EAT
WELL
LOOK
GREAT

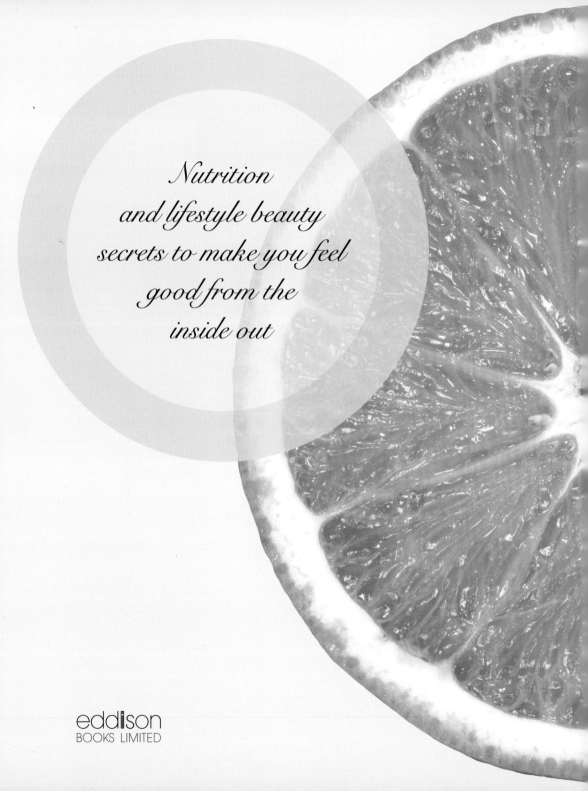

*Nutrition
and lifestyle beauty
secrets to make you feel
good from the
inside out*

eddison
BOOKS LIMITED

EAT
WELL

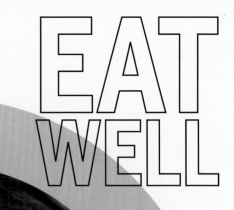

LOOK
GREAT

Dr Sarah Brewer

*This book is dedicated to my wonderful family,
who willingly provided invaluable back-up and support
during those long hours of research and writing.*

This edition published in Great Britain in 2018 by
Eddison Books Limited
St Chad's House, 148 King's Cross Road
London WC1X 9DH
www.eddisonbooks.com

British Library Cataloguing-in-Publication data available on request.

ISBN 978-1-85906-398-9

10 9 8 7 6 5 4 3 2 1

Phototypeset in Benton Gothic, Life and Snell Roundhand
using InDesign on Apple Macintosh
Printed in China

CONTENTS

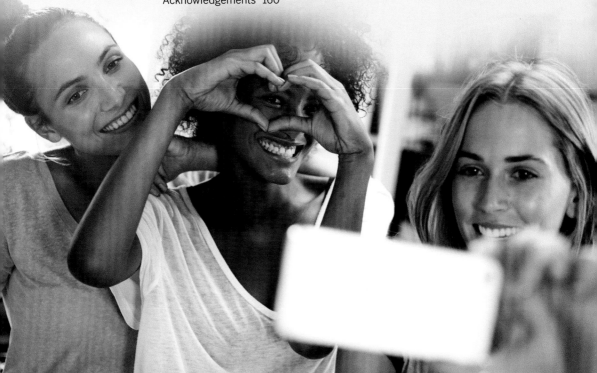

INTRODUCTION

Throughout the ages, women have sought a variety of ways to accentuate and retain their beauty. Cleopatra bathed in Dead Sea mineral mud and asses' milk, while the fashionistas in Ancient Rome used lead salts to whiten their complexion. But beauty is more than just skin deep; good nutrition is one of the best-kept beauty secrets for staving off wrinkles and maintaining youthfulness.

How nutrition and beauty are linked

Your skin, hair and nails are formed by cells that are among the most rapidly dividing in your body, and therefore need a constant supply of nutrients for optimum health. As a result, they are often the first areas to show signs of nutritional deficiencies. Key nutrients that are in short supply are preferentially absorbed and used by other vital tissues, such as the brain, thyroid, bone marrow and liver, leaving your skin, hair and nails to fend for themselves.

During times of stress, when the body goes into 'fight or flight' mode, stress hormones such as adrenaline and cortisol also divert blood away from your hair, skin and nails towards your muscles (for running or fighting) and your brain (to help you think more quickly). This diversion of the circulation reduces the supply of oxygen, glucose and micronutrients to your rapidly dividing hair, skin and nails.

A reduced blood supply, or poor nutrition, also reduces your supply of dietary antioxidants and oestrogen-like plant hormones, which are the closest thing we currently have to an elixir of life to slow the ageing process in these tissues. Antioxidants, for example, help to neutralize the free radicals (unstable molecules that can damage cells) that trigger age spots, loss of skin elasticity, wrinkles and thinning hair. Researchers have found that antioxidants can reduce skin roughness and improve skin tone, clarity and radiance, while reducing fine wrinkles and overall aged appearance.

Plant oestrogens, such as soy isoflavones and lignans found in nuts, seeds and vegetables like pumpkin and sweet potato, provide a useful hormone boost in older women whose own oestrogen production is falling. Oestrogen helps to regulate collagen production in the skin, and good dietary intakes help to reduce some of the visible signs of ageing.

Essential fatty acids found in evening primrose, flaxseed, fish and nut oils are also important for healthy, flexible cell membranes, helping your skin stay moist, strengthening nails and improving the glossiness of your hair.

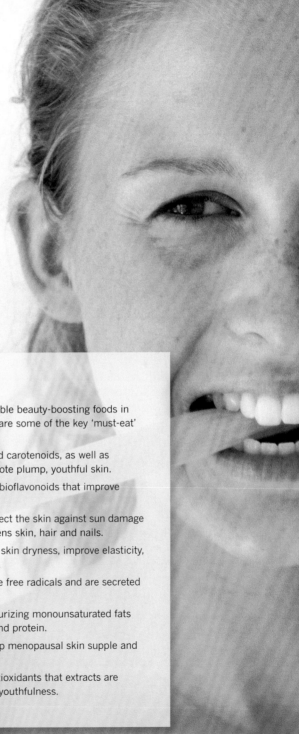

TAKING ACTION

All of this means that the key to looking and feeling great is really in your hands: only *you* can provide the right kind of nutritional fuel to give your body what it needs to function at – and look – its best. And this book reveals the secrets to help you do just that.

Together with the lifestyle advice given on the pages that follow, plus the tailored lifestyle tips, recipes and guidance on useful supplements and salon therapies featured throughout the book, you have all the knowledge you need at your fingertips. It's time to take matters into your own hands – and discover how feeling good *inside* can help you look good *outside*. (NOTE: All recipes included in the book serve four, unless otherwise stated.)

TOP BEAUTY-BOOSTING FOODS

You'll be finding out more about the most valuable beauty-boosting foods in Part 1 of the book (see pages 20–87), but here are some of the key 'must-eat' favourites:

Avocado supplies antioxidant vitamins C, E and carotenoids, as well as moisturizing monounsaturated fats which promote plump, youthful skin.

Berries are excellent sources of vitamin C and bioflavonoids that improve collagen formation and help keep skin supple.

Carrots contain carotenoids, which help to protect the skin against sun damage and are a good source of silica, which strengthens skin, hair and nails.

Fish provide omega-3 fatty acids, which reduce skin dryness, improve elasticity, strengthen nails and add a glossy sheen to hair.

Garlic contains sulphur compounds that reduce free radicals and are secreted directly onto the skin via sweat glands.

Macadamia nut oil is a richer source of moisturizing monounsaturated fats than olive oil, and a good source of vitamin E and protein.

Soy beans provide isoflavones that help to keep menopausal skin supple and combat dryness and wrinkles.

Green tea is so full of anti-ageing flavonoid antioxidants that extracts are now being added to cosmetics to improve skin youthfulness.

LIVING SENSIBLY

Sun exposure

When ultraviolet rays strike your skin, they generate free radicals and an inflammatory reaction known as heliodermatitis. UVB rays are associated with sunburn and some signs of skin ageing, but the worst culprits are UVA rays, which make up 95 per cent of ultraviolet wavelengths. These penetrate more deeply into your skin and can even pass through glass, so you are exposed when sitting by an office window or in a car.

UV rays damage skin structures, interfere with normal cell division and activate enzymes that dissolve skin proteins. As a result, collagen and elastin fibres become increasingly thick, twisted and cross-linked. At the same time, a substance called hyaluronan, which attracts water into your skin, decreases, so your skin loses its resilience and elasticity. Small veins dilate to form visible red lines, and poor circulation leads to a sallow, dull complexion. Dark age spots develop, along with mottling and white areas of depigmentation. In extreme cases, skin becomes highly wrinkled, yellow and mottled, with a coarse, pebbly, leathery texture.

Every time your skin is exposed to the sun it's damaged by ultraviolet rays. Over the years, this damage adds up, leading to premature wrinkles (pages 98–9), skin blemishes and age spots (pages 96–7). Excessive sun exposure is also linked with an increased risk of skin cancer.

IDENTIFYING AGE SPOTS

Age spots are patches of skin discoloration commonly seen on the backs of the hands, face and neck. There are five main types:

- irregular mottling due to changes in skin pigment cells
- white, star-shaped false scars that tend to appear after the age of sixty
- small, pure white round or angular spots
- small brown marks which darken in the sun
- darkened patches of skin that can be over 1 cm (½ in) across and which are often dark brown, but may also be yellow, light brown or even black

SUN PROTECTION AND VITAMIN D

Wearing sunscreen is one of the most effective ways to reduce premature skin ageing, if any part of your skin will be exposed to the sun for more than 20 minutes. Some sun exposure is important, however, to synthesize vitamin D in the body. Vitamin D is involved in regulating the production of hair, skin and nails, though you can only synthesize it when the UV index is above 3 (so this is subject to seasonal and regional variation). Just 15 minutes' sun exposure is sufficient to meet our vitamin D needs. Vitamin D is also obtained in the diet from oily fish, eggs, butter and fortified milk.

Lifestyle checklist

- Use a high protection factor sunscreen (at least SPF15) even during winter. Select products that also protect against UVA.
- Avoid going in the sun between 11am and 2pm, when the sun's rays are strongest.
- Cover up with loose, light clothing – you can still burn on hazy days, and even in the shade.
- Tan slowly with a maximum of 20–30 minutes' exposure on the first day, then build up slowly by no more than 5 minutes per day.
- Don't forget to protect sensitive areas such as your nose, nipples, soles of feet, ears and the top of your head – especially if you're balding. A knotted handkerchief is better than nothing if you don't have a wide-brimmed hat!
- Use a waterproof sunscreen if you are swimming, and reapply as soon as you come out of the water.
- Keep your skin well moisturized before and after sunbathing to prevent it from drying out.
- Take extra care on the beach – the flat surface of the water can reflect 100 per cent of UV rays back up at you, while sand can reflect up to 20 per cent of UV rays.
- Protect your eyes by only wearing sunglasses bearing the BSI mark (or regional equivalent).
- Make sure babies and children are well protected with sunblock creams, cover-up clothing and sun hats, as much of the UV damage associated with premature skin ageing occurs during childhood.

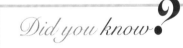

Did you know?

A diet that is rich in the antioxidant vitamins C, E and betacarotene (found in yellow-orange fruit and vegetables such as papaya, carrots, pumpkin and sweet potato) helps to protect against some of the damaging effects of the sun's rays. Lycopene, a red carotenoid pigment found in papaya, guava, pink grapefruit, watermelon and tomato, also protects your skin from the ageing effects of UV light.

Beauty sleep

Sleep is a natural time of regeneration and rejuvenation. It is when growth hormone is secreted to direct and speed the repair of ageing tissues and maintain the collagen matrix that keeps tissues plump and reduces wrinkling. When you achieve a good night's sleep, you feel energized during the day, find it easier to concentrate and cope with stress, and also appear more attractive. Research published in the *British Medical Journal* in which untrained observers were shown photographs of people who had either slept for 8 hours or had been awake for 31 hours found that those who were sleep-deprived were perceived as less healthy, less attractive and more tired than those who'd had a normal night's sleep. It may seem obvious, but getting sufficient sleep reduces puffiness and bags around the eyes, helps to prevent dark circles beneath the eyes and avoids redness. It also helps your skin to glow.

Another study from the University of Birmingham, UK, found that, when sleep is restricted to 4 hours per night, blood vessels throughout the body – including the skin – are less able to dilate. At the same time, tired people breathe more shallowly so blood oxygen levels decrease. This, in turn, reduces the delivery of vitamins, minerals and oxygen to your skin, hair and nails, as well as reducing the flushing away of toxins and carbon dioxide. Unsurprisingly, this has a knock-on effect on your looks. Tiredness makes your skin appear washed out, pale and lacking lustre. Never underestimate the value of a good night's beauty sleep!

If you feel tired during the day, try taking a power nap: short naps of 5–15 minutes are proven to have a significant effect at promoting energy renewal. A power nap involves

Lifestyle checklist

- Avoid eating large or spicy meals during the evening, as the digestive process can inhibit deep sleep.
- Don't drink tea, coffee or any drink containing caffeine for at least 3 hours before your normal bedtime.
- Sprinkle a few drops of lavender essential oil on a cotton-wool pad near your pillow, or invest in a lavender-scented pillow; inhaling this natural sedative oil can help you relax and improves sleep.
- Have a bath containing Dead Sea mineral salts before going to bed. These contain magnesium, which is absorbed through the skin for a muscle-relaxing effect that promotes sleep.
- Avoid vigorous exercise in the evening, as this will have an alerting effect (regular exercise during the day is still important).
- Use eyelash curlers, if all else fails! These will make your eyes appear more open and awake, especially when teamed with lengthening mascara to widen your eyes.

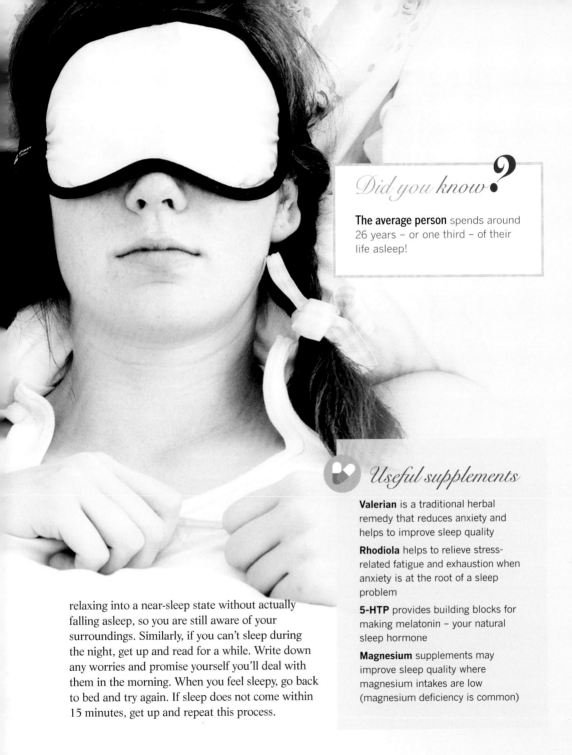

Did you know?

The average person spends around 26 years – or one third – of their life asleep!

Useful supplements

Valerian is a traditional herbal remedy that reduces anxiety and helps to improve sleep quality

Rhodiola helps to relieve stress-related fatigue and exhaustion when anxiety is at the root of a sleep problem

5-HTP provides building blocks for making melatonin – your natural sleep hormone

Magnesium supplements may improve sleep quality where magnesium intakes are low (magnesium deficiency is common)

relaxing into a near-sleep state without actually falling asleep, so you are still aware of your surroundings. Similarly, if you can't sleep during the night, get up and read for a while. Write down any worries and promise yourself you'll deal with them in the morning. When you feel sleepy, go back to bed and try again. If sleep does not come within 15 minutes, get up and repeat this process.

One of the best ways to revitalize dull skin is to go for a brisk 20-minute walk. The combination of exercise, fresh air, deeper breathing and exposure to sunlight will impart a healthy glow.

Exercise

Taking regular exercise can prolong your life – and help to improve your looks. Exercise has a dynamic effect on your circulation, boosting blood flow to your hair, skin and nails to increase the delivery of oxygen, vitamins, minerals, plant oestrogens and other phytonutrients.

And that's not all. As well as improving your strength, stamina and suppleness, regular exercise helps you maintain a healthy weight, improves digestion and reduces anxiety and tension, in addition to helping you sleep more deeply. Exercise also firms muscles and improves lymph drainage, to clear a build-up of waste products from tissues. This helps to prevent or reduce cellulite, as well as firming your silhouette. Find an exercise you enjoy, such as dancing, cycling or yoga (inversion or upside-down yoga poses are also good for stimulating the growth of healthy hair).

Raising a sweat is also good for the hair, skin and nails. It helps to speed the flushing of cellular wastes and debris, and normalizes the production of skin oils, to reduce oiliness as well as combating dryness. In addition, sweating boosts the secretion of salt and reduces fluid retention. A good workout therefore helps to reduce eye puffiness and dark circles. And, by reducing levels of cortisol hormone, exercise helps you relax and promotes a good night's sleep.

BEAT STRESS – BEAT WRINKLES

Exercise is one of the best ways to burn off the effects of stress hormones, as it switches the 'fight or flight' reaction back to the 'rest and digest' response, just as nature intended. It also promotes secretion of soothing brain chemicals such as serotonin, dopamine and endorphins to perk you up and help you feel better. Less stress means fewer frown lines, while feeling happy helps you radiate a positive, beautiful glow as you smile.

Research from the University of California found that cells from stressed women who exercised vigorously, for around 42 minutes per day, showed fewer changes associated with premature ageing and wrinkles than a similar group of stressed women who did not exercise. What's more, these changes were seen within just three days.

Did you know?

According to the *Journal of the American Dental Association*, people who exercise are up to 40 per cent less likely to develop gum disease and have better oral health than non-exercisers. Improved circulation is thought to deliver essential nutrients to teeth and gums, helping you to retain an attractive smile.

Alcohol

Did you know?

1 unit of alcohol (10 g) is equivalent to each of the following:
- 300 ml ($^1/_2$ pt) beer
- 100 ml (3$^1/_2$ fl oz) wine (10 per cent alcohol by volume)
- 50 ml (1$^3/_4$ fl oz) sherry
- 25 ml (1 fl oz) spirits

While a small amount of alcohol has a relaxing effect, which can be beneficial in reducing stress, an excess intake is harmful to both your health and your looks. Alcohol is a cell poison which can damage the cells renewing your skin, hair and nails to reduce their quality, leading to dry, patchy hair loss, dull, dry skin and weak, brittle nails. In addition, excess alcohol lowers female oestrogen levels, which can lead to premature ageing with wrinkles, patchy skin pigmentation and thinning hair.

Drinking excess alcohol depletes the body of nutrients that are rapidly used up during its metabolism. These include vitamin C, which is needed to make collagen in the skin, and B group vitamins, which are important for healthy hair, skin and nails. Alcohol also contributes to weight gain, as it provides more energy, per gram, than either protein or carbohydrate, delivering as much as 7 kcal per gram in addition to the sugars that are normally also present in wine and mixers to provide sweetness.

Another important factor to consider when drinking alcohol is that, although it may initially cause drowsiness so you quickly fall asleep, it interferes with sleep architecture, so you are likely to wake and have a disturbed night once the drug effect wears off. This causes disrupted rest, as does its diuretic action, which may cause you to wake to visit the bathroom in the night. Dehydration and lack of sleep means you are likely to wake with puffy eyes, dark circles, red-rimmed eyes and tired, sallow skin – not an attractive look!

Lifestyle checklist
- Drink plenty of fluids – alternate alcoholic with non-alcoholic drinks.
- Mix wine half-and-half with sparkling water for a refreshing spritzer.
- Rehydrate with freshly squeezed orange juice, which supplies vitamin C as well as fluid.
- Offer to be the designated driver on a night out, and drink fresh-fruit-juice mocktails for a vitamin boost, on the house.

Smoking

If you smoke, do your utmost to stop. The harmful chemicals present in cigarette smoke damage cells throughout the body. As well as increasing the risk of just about every type of cancer, this leads to widespread premature ageing effects. In skin, this shows up as premature wrinkles, which usually appear first in the delicate skin around the eyes to produce a tell-tale bagginess. Vertical wrinkles also appear around the mouth where skin is pursed through the physical act of clamping a cigarette between the lips. Skin tone also becomes dull through lack of oxygen and may appear pale or develop uneven colouring, and teeth and tongue may become discoloured with nicotine.

Smoking-related wrinkles appear within a few years and become more numerous and pronounced the longer you smoke. Ongoing studies involving identical twins, one of whom smokes and one who doesn't, show dramatic differences, with the smoking twin often looking at least ten years older than their sibling – and often old enough to be their parent.

Smoking leads to wrinkles through a number of different mechanisms. Over 4,000 chemicals are present in tobacco smoke. These damage collagen and elastin, which give skin its strength and elasticity, and lower vitamin C levels so there is less available for production of new collagen. Smoking causes narrowing and spasm of blood vessels supplying the hair, skin and nails, reducing blood flow and the delivery of oxygen and nutrients – especially the all-important antioxidants such as vitamins A, C and E.

Smoking has also been shown to reduce oestrogen levels, so that, on average, female smokers experience the menopause two years earlier than non-smokers. All these factors combined add up to a beauty no-no.

QUIT PLAN

- **Find support** – stopping smoking is easier if you do it with a friend or relative.
- **Name the day to give up** and get into the right frame of mind.
- **Throw away all cigarettes,** matches, lighters and ashtrays.
- **Take it one day at a time** – keep a chart and tick off each cigarette-free day.
- **Occupy your hands** by drawing, writing, model-making, painting, knitting, or doing embroidery, DIY or even origami.
- **Exercise briskly** to help curb withdrawal symptoms.
- **Avoid situations where you used to smoke.**

Electronic cigarettes, nicotine replacement therapy and medication are available to help you cut back, if you would find that easier than going 'cold turkey'. Seek advice from your doctor or a pharmacist.

Adding lime juice to food stimulates taste buds and decreases the amount of salt you need.

Salt

Common table salt – known chemically as sodium chloride – is added to many foods to enhance flavour, retain moisture and lengthen shelf life. Only a small amount of salt is needed to maintain healthy cells, however – estimated at just over 1 g per day. Many people consume nine times this amount or more! When you consume salt, most of the sodium is kept outside your cells in exchange for potassium, which is pumped inside cells. Any excess sodium therefore builds up in the fluid bathing your cells – known as your internal sea – where it, in turn, attracts a build-up of fluid to keep it dissolved.

Lifestyle checklist

To cut back on salt intake, avoid:

- adding salt during cooking or at the table
- obviously salty foods such as crisps, bacon, salted nuts
- tinned products, especially those canned in brine
- cured, smoked or pickled fish/meats
- meat pastes, pâtés
- ready-prepared meals
- packet soups and sauces
- stock cubes and yeast extracts

Some people have kidneys that are efficient at excreting the excess salt and fluid, but many people do not. As a result, the retained salt and its accompanying fluid can lead to puffiness, especially around the eyes. It also increases your blood pressure. For women, the hormone fluctuations associated with the menstrual cycle can cause fluid fluctuations equivalent to retaining 1–2 kg (around 2–4 lb) weight at certain times of the month.

WATCH YOUR INTAKE

Traditionally, the majority of dietary salt was adding during cooking and at the table. Now, 75 per cent of dietary salt is obtained from processed foods, including canned products, ready-prepared meals, biscuits, cakes and breakfast cereals. Some foods are 30 per cent more salty than sea water, which contains 2.5 g salt per 100 g water.

Always check the labels of bought products, and avoid those containing high amounts of salt. A good general rule is that, per 100 g (3½ oz) food (or per serving, if a serving is less than 100 g): 0.5 g sodium (1.25 g salt) or more is *a lot* of sodium; 0.1 g sodium (0.25 g salt) or less is *a little* sodium. NOTE: To convert 'sodium' to salt content, simply multiply by 2.5 – so, for example, 0.4 g sodium is equivalent to 1 g salt (sodium chloride).

Salt can be replaced with herbs and spices such as black pepper for flavour. When cutting back on salt it takes around a month to retrain your taste buds; food may taste bland initially until your taste buds learn to respond to lower salt concentrations. When essential, use a low-sodium, high-potassium salt, or mineral-rich rock or sea salt rather than table salt, and use sparingly. Potassium helps to flush excess sodium and fluid from the body via the kidneys; good sources include seafood, fresh fruit, vegetables, juices and wholegrains.

Water: the importance of hydration

Water is one of the most important beauty-boosting nutrients in your diet. It is essential for plump skin, delivery of nutrients to hair and nail-building cells, and for flushing away wastes.

You normally maintain a fine fluid balance which is regulated partly by hormonal control and partly by the concentration of salts, sugars and soluble proteins in your circulation. As long as you replace your daily water losses through adequate drinking and eating, you will avoid dehydration and help to maintain plump, healthy skin and bright, beautiful eyes, while avoiding dry, brittle hair and nails. For most women, that means obtaining 2 to 3 litres (4 to 6 pints) per day from drinks and moisture-rich foods such as soups, yogurt, fruit and vegetables.

Dehydration is a common cause of tiredness, poor concentration, reduced alertness, reduced short-term memory, headache and mood changes. It also increases the stickiness of blood, and reduces the delivery of oxygen and nutrients to your cells. When you are dehydrated, your skin loses its attractive glow, and gives you a tired, haggard appearance with more pronounced sagging and dullness. Blood vessels in the thin skin beneath the eyes may become more visible, leading to dark circles.

BOTTLED OR TAP? SPARKLING OR STILL?

Tap water is treated to remove harmful substances (such as agricultural contaminants) and disinfected with chlorine. Placing a covered jug of water in the fridge until it is cool (around an hour) will help to remove chlorine traces (use within 24 hours). Using a water filter will also remove chlorine and improve flavour. Table water, offered by some restaurants at a high price, is often just bottled tap water that has been filtered to improve its taste.

Spring water may be treated to remove certain minerals or undesirable substances, but its composition does not have to be specified. In contrast, mineral water is bottled at a single, identified and protected source, with a guaranteed consistent composition, and, by definition, has not undergone any treatments. Both are available as still or sparkling.

All types of water will help to maintain hydration, so it's just down to personal taste as to which you prefer.

Did you know?

Water makes up around 55 per cent of the weight of an average female, while in males this increases to around 60 per cent, due to the lower relative amount of body fat present.

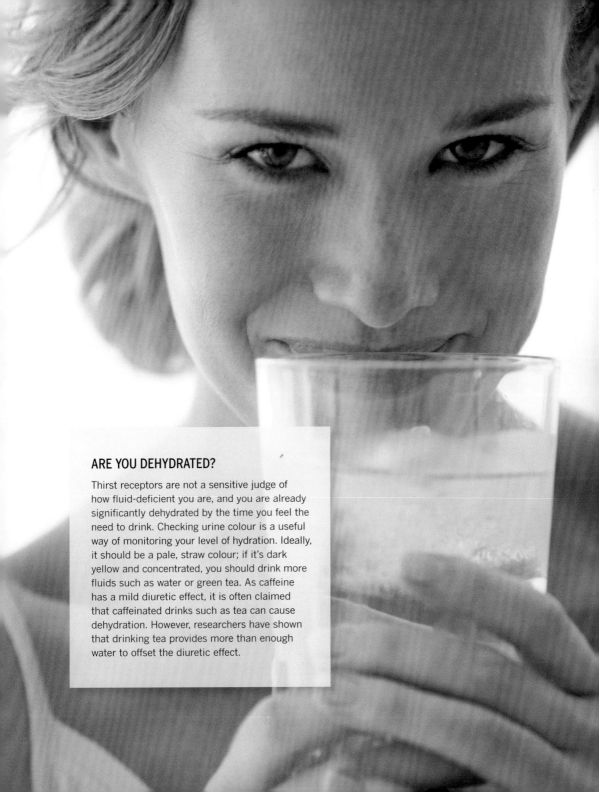

ARE YOU DEHYDRATED?

Thirst receptors are not a sensitive judge of how fluid-deficient you are, and you are already significantly dehydrated by the time you feel the need to drink. Checking urine colour is a useful way of monitoring your level of hydration. Ideally, it should be a pale, straw colour; if it's dark yellow and concentrated, you should drink more fluids such as water or green tea. As caffeine has a mild diuretic effect, it is often claimed that caffeinated drinks such as tea can cause dehydration. However, researchers have shown that drinking tea provides more than enough water to offset the diuretic effect.

Reducing acidity in your diet

Water ionizes to produce hydrogen ions (H^+ or protons) and hydroxyl ions (OH^-). Because the protons and hydroxyl ions are present in equal proportions, the acidity of water is considered neutral with a pH of 7. Fluids with a higher concentration of protons are acidic (pH below 7) while fluids with a higher concentration of hydroxyl ions are alkaline (pH between 7 and 14).

Each pH unit of difference represents a tenfold difference in concentration, as the pH scale is logarithmic. So, a liquid with a pH of 5 is ten times more acidic than a liquid with a pH of 6, and one hundred times more acidic than water with a pH of 7.

Your body works hard to keep your blood and the fluids bathing your cells within a very tight pH range of 7.35 to 7.45, which is slightly alkaline. Even slight movements outside of this narrow pH range will severely affect your cells, changing the three-dimensional shapes of cell proteins and enzymes, and affecting nerve messages and muscle contraction.

ACID OR ALKALINE?

Most of the acid in your body is ultimately derived from your diet and the processing of the proteins, carbohydrates and fats it provides. If the metabolism of a food results in the production of excess protons, it's classified as an acid-forming food. If the metabolism of a food uses up more protons than it produces, however, it's classified as an alkaline-forming food. This classification is based on the effect a food has after it has been processed, and whether or not it raises or lowers the acidity (pH) of your urine; it is not based on whether the food itself is acidic or alkaline in quality.

Many acid-tasting foods such as lemons, oranges and tomatoes actually have an alkaline effect on the body. This may seem confusing, but is because the fruit acids present (such as citric acid and malic acid) are weak acids and do not break down to release protons (H^+) to any great extent. Instead, they are readily neutralized by the large amount of potassium also present in the fruit to form salts such as potassium citrate and potassium malate. During metabolism, these salts react with sodium, water and carbon dioxide in your cells to form sodium bicarbonate, which has an alkaline effect on urine. Adding sugar to fruit juices reduces the buffering effect of potassium, however, so sweetened fruit juices become acid-forming.

Protein-rich foods such as meat and dairy products are the main acid-forming foods in your diet, even though they don't taste acidic when you eat them. This is because the amino acids they contain are broken down to produce excess protons, which acidify your urine. Normally, your body processes acid-forming foods without undue difficulty. However, many nutritionists recommend following a relatively alkaline diet and avoiding excess acid-forming foods, to decrease the level of inflammation in the body. This is believed to help combat premature ageing, improve immune function, and promote healthy hair, skin and nails.

Did you know?

Many carbonated soft drinks have a pH of 3, making them 10,000 times more acid than water (pH 7).

GET THE BALANCE RIGHT

For optimal beauty benefits, aim to eat a balanced diet that consists of 60–80 per cent alkaline foods and only 20–40 per cent acid foods. Essentially, this means eating more fruit and green leafy vegetables and cutting back on the amount of animal proteins and processed foods you eat, while still maintaining a regular intake of protein. Eat animal proteins (eggs, poultry, meats, seafood) no more than once a day and make sure you have regular vegetarian days, too.

Aim to consume more alkaline-forming foods:
green tea • tomatoes • berries • grapefruit • figs • peppers • some pulses (alfalfa, lentils, lima beans, soy beans, navy beans) • some nuts (almonds, pine nuts, chestnuts) • sweet potato • squash/pumpkin • parsnips • artichokes • courgettes • aubergines • green leafy vegetables (kale, broccoli, spinach, barley grass, wheat grass) • coconut • sour cherries • mango • apricots • ripe bananas • dates • melon • watermelon • herbs (parsley, coriander leaf, oregano) • avocado • celery • asparagus • green beans • beetroot • radish • garlic

Maintain a balanced intake of mildly acid-forming foods:
vegetables with a high protein or sulphur content (such as peas, sweetcorn, cauliflower, cabbage, leeks, asparagus, onions); grains (barley, oats, quinoa, rice, wheat, flours, bread, pasta) • some pulses (such as black beans, chickpeas, kidney beans) • some nuts (pecans, cashews, peanuts, pistachios, walnuts) • dairy products (cream, cheese, milk, ice cream) • wine • apple cider vinegar • sparkling water • vegetable oils

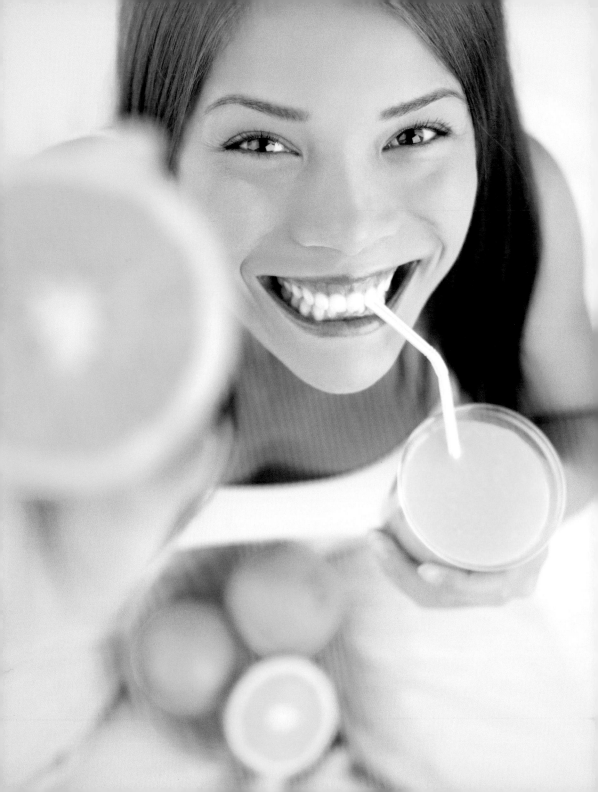

1

Beauty-Boosting Superfoods

Discover the beauty benefits of forty superfoods to
incorporate in your everyday beauty regime,
to make you feel – and look – fantastic.

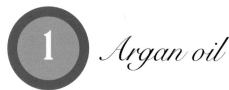

1 *Argan oil*

Oil from the Moroccan argan tree (*Argania spinosa*) has been used for centuries as a health and beauty treatment. It is often referred to as 'liquid gold', thanks to its skin rejuvenating, plumping and nourishing qualities.

Interest and research into argan oil's benefits in recent years mean it is now one of the most prized oils in the world. It is a rich source of antioxidants, vitamin E, essential fatty acids, squalene and phytosterols, and is produced in three grades:

- **virgin beauty argan oil**, prepared from unroasted nuts which are cracked and the inner kernels ground into a paste to extract the oil (one tree, producing 30 kg/66 lb of fruit, delivers just 1 litre/2 pints of oil per year, which is why it is so expensive). The oil has a pale golden colour, no flavour and a unique, light smell
- **virgin edible argan oil**, pressed from kernels that have been lightly roasted over a low flame for a few minutes to enhance the distinctive argan oil flavour and achieve a deeper, copper colour
- **cosmetic argan oil**, prepared by solvent extraction and used in shampoos, moisturizers and other cosmetic products

Caution

Argan oil is a traditional treatment for problem skin and should not sting when applied. However, a few cases of allergic contact dermatitis have been reported, so patch-test a small area of skin before use.

Buying tip

Choose products labelled as 100 per cent argan oil or *Argania spinosa* kernel oil, sold in dark-coloured glass (often amber or cobalt blue), aluminium or stainless steel containers, because light quickly deteriorates argan oil stored in clear or plastic bottles.

On the inside

The total antioxidant capacity of virgin argan oil is higher than that of other vegetable oils, and researchers have confirmed that its consumption significantly raises blood vitamin E levels in postmenopausal women. This contributes to beneficial effects on liver function, cholesterol balance, blood pressure and glucose control, as well as its reputation for reducing premature skin ageing.

Argan oil is a natural source of melatonin, a hormone that promotes sleep. By helping to ensure a good night's rest, argan oil can help you achieve a fresher look with less pronounced bags and dark circles beneath the eyes.

In your diet Argan oil adds a characteristic, lightly toasted nutty flavour to tagines, and is delicious sprinkled on salads, roast vegetables or grilled goat's cheese, or stirred into soups, pasta or couscous. Use sparingly and add after cooking to preserve its health benefits. (Do not use for frying.)

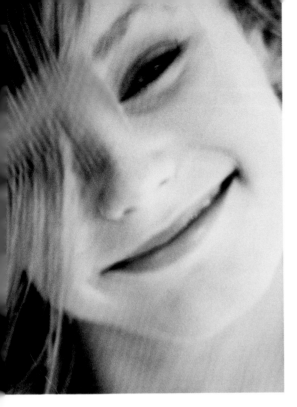

with acne or dandruff, and also reduces the synthesis of melanin, to improve hyperpigmentation.

Interestingly, in addition to having a moisturizing effect on dry skin, it is equally good for oily skin, as it helps to normalize the production of skin oil (sebum). It can even be used as a base under make-up due to its non-oily nature; in tests on volunteers with oily facial skin, twice-daily use for four weeks significantly reduced greasiness in appearance. Studies in postmenopausal women have also shown that, applied daily, argan oil significantly reduced water loss from the skin to improve hydration within two months.

When applied to hair, it strengthens protein bonds, improves elasticity and restores smoothness and lustre, giving new life to dry, tangled, flyaway strands. It also protect against heat treatments such as blow-drying.

On the outside

Argan oil is applied neat to the skin, hair and nails, or combined with other ingredients in luxury skincare ranges. It boasts moisturizing, wound-healing, anti-scarring and anti-ageing properties, and is used to treat dry skin, acne, psoriasis, eczema, wrinkles, inflamed skin and painful joints. It feels smooth and silky, and is easily absorbed without leaving a sticky residue.

As well as protecting skin from environmental damage, its antioxidants help to prevent the breakdown of elastin and collagen – the structural proteins maintaining skin plumpness and elasticity – to reduce stretch marks, fine lines and wrinkles. It soothes dry, sensitive skin and damps down inflammation associated

Beauty secrets
● Gently massage it into your scalp and hair to hydrate, protect and nourish follicles, and to tame dry, frizzy or damaged hair, restoring its natural shine.
● Place a few drops on your brush or comb to give your hair freshness, brilliance and lustre.
● Use to soak your cuticles to keep them soft and promote the growth of stronger, less brittle nails.
● Make a lip scrub to soften dry lips by mixing a few drops of argan oil with brown sugar, and gently massaging it in.
● Add a few drops to your moisturizer or foundation for a naturally rehydrated glow.
● Mix a few drops with pure rose water for a refreshing skin toner.
● Put a few drops into your bath water for a rejuvenating soak.

2 *Coconut oil*

This **wonderful oil**, with its characteristic fragrance, is a health and beauty essential in the tropics. As well as being used in the kitchen, it's a popular hair and skin moisturizer with antiseptic properties.

On the inside

Although coconut oil consists of over 90 per cent saturated fats, these are mostly in the form of medium-chain fatty acids such as lauric acid and caprylic acid, which offer many health benefits. They are used by the liver as a fuel rather than being stored as fat, and boost liver function to speed the metabolic rate so you burn up to three times more calories for 6 hours after a meal than when consuming other vegetable oils (which contain long-chain triglycerides). In one study, volunteers consuming four to five teaspoons of coconut oil per day in baked goods and cooked meals lost, over a four-month period, nearly 2 kg (4 lb) more than subjects who used the same amount of olive oil.

Coconut oil fatty acids also have a natural antiviral, antibacterial and anti-

---

Did you know?

Coconut water from green coconuts is a great beauty drink, as it's hydrating, relatively low in calories and enriched with electrolytes such as potassium and magnesium, which help to reduce blood pressure.

---

fungal action that inhibits Candida yeasts, for example, which can cause thrush and fungal skin infections.

In your diet Use it for all types of cooking, baking and frying (the oil can withstand high temperatures), or try stirring a spoon into yogurt, smoothies or hot drinks for a delicious rich taste.

On the outside

Research shows that coconut oil creams significantly improve skin elasticity, smoothness and tone, reducing the appearance of fine lines and wrinkles. Recent studies also suggest virgin coconut oil can boost wound-healing, by reducing water loss and making it easier for new skin cells to 'leapfrog' over one another into the healing area.

A study on adults with xerosis – characterized by dry, rough, scaly and itchy skin – found that applying coconut oil as a moisturizer twice a day for two weeks significantly improved skin hydration and strengthened its lipid barrier. It's also safe to use on infants and children: applying virgin coconut oil was found to significantly improve symptoms in seven out of ten children suffering from eczema in one study, with almost half showing an excellent response.

Unlike mineral oils, coconut oil is rich in lauric acid, which has a high affinity for hair proteins. It penetrates deeply into hair shafts, without disrupting its natural scale structure, and leaves a thinner film on the surface than other oils. Coconut oil treatments are particularly useful for preventing hair damage during combing.

Beauty secrets

- **Apply as a night cream** to smooth fine lines and wrinkles.
- **Use on a cotton-wool ball** to cleanse your face and remove make-up – including waterproof mascara and eyeshadow.
- **Highlight your cheeks** with a little oil for a healthy sheen.
- **Use as a lip balm** for dry, chapped lips (though avoid strong sun, as it only has a natural sun protection factor of around 4).
- **Massage into dry hands** as a soothing moisturizer that also nourishes cuticles.
- **Apply to wet skin** as a body oil after a shower or bath, then pat dry to smell wonderful all day. Pay special attention to dry, itchy areas.
- **Smooth a tiny amount onto hair ends** as a leave-in conditioner, to add shine and tame frizziness. (When holidaying in the tropics, coconut oil helps to protect your hair from the drying effects of the sun.)
- **Massage a tablespoon of oil** into your scalp, then gently comb through your hair, for deep, overnight conditioning. Cover with a shower cap, wrap your hair in a warm towel turban for at least an hour, or overnight, then shampoo as usual. This is a great natural treatment for dandruff.
- **Use as a shaving cream** for legs or underarms – it moisturizes the skin and helps the blade glide.
- **Use a spoonful** as a mouth rinse, swilling it round and 'pulling' it through your teeth to cleanse your gums and freshen your breath.

MAKE A BODY SCRUB:

Combine melted coconut oil with demerara sugar or coarse sea salt, stirring well. Massage all over the body, paying attention to dry areas such as elbows, knees and heels.

3 *Evening primrose oil*

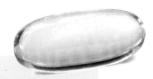

The beautiful evening primrose flower blooms for just one day, but its oil helps your skin bloom year after year. It is a rich source of an essential fatty acid called GLA; lack of essential fatty acids has been linked with dry, itchy skin, acne, brittle hair and nails and hair loss.

FOR A TOPICAL TREATMENT:

Pierce a capsule of evening primrose oil and apply to dry areas of skin.

On the inside

Evening primrose oil (EPO) is one of the most popular and useful food supplements, as up to 10 per cent of its essential fatty acid content is GLA (gamma linolenic or gamolenic acid) – one of the few omega-6 oils with an anti-inflammatory action similar to that of omega-3s, when intakes are sufficiently high. (Other sources include blackcurrant seed oil and starflower, or borage, oil.)

Some GLA is incorporated into cell membranes, making them more flexible. In the skin, this produces a noticeable improvement in softness and hydration within a few days. Some is also converted into hormone-like substances known as series 1 prostaglandins, which relax blood vessels to improve blood flow to the skin, decrease inflammation to reduce redness,

and improve nerve function to reduce itching and discomfort. It may also have a beneficial effect on hormone balance to improve the severity of hot flushes and dry skin at the menopause. In fact, the folk name for evening primrose is 'King's cure-all', as it offers so many health benefits.

Although your cells produce small amounts of GLA, this process is easily blocked by factors such as increasing age, smoking, pollution, lack of certain vitamins and minerals and excessive intakes of saturated fat, sugar or alcohol, so deficiency is common. When lacking in essential fatty acids, your skin becomes scaly, rough, itchy, prematurely wrinkled and feels dry. Paradoxically, it also becomes more prone to spots, as oil gland ducts become distorted and trap grease. Here are just some of the ways that EPO can help:

Maintain skin hydration EPO helps to stabilize the skin barrier, to maintain hydration when taken either as capsules or applied as a water-in-oil emulsion. A review of nine studies found that it frequently reduced the symptoms of dry itchy skin/eczema after several months' use, with a significant reduction in itching.

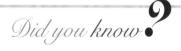

Did you know?

When combined with fish oils, the beneficial anti-inflammatory effects of EPO are increased – so boost your intake of omega-3s.

Soften skin EPO helps make skin softer, providing a more youthful appearance. In one trial involving women in their forties, those taking 3 g evening primrose oil experienced a 20 per cent improvement in skin moisture, smoothness, elasticity and firmness within three months.

Improve skin luminosity In the laboratory, EPO has been shown to reduce over-production of the pigment melanin in skin cells. It appears to work by reducing the activity of an enzyme (tyrosinase) involved in melanin synthesis. Topical application of EPO is a potential cosmetic whitening agent to reduce mottled or patchy skin.

Reduce dry eyes – especially in contact-lens wearers. A study involving women who took either EPO or placebo (olive oil) for six months found those taking EPO showed significant improvement in dryness and overall lens comfort. The viscosity of tears was also increased.

Evening primrose oil can help reduce eye dryness in contact-lens wearers.

On the outside

Evening primrose oil is regularly used in anti-ageing creams, thanks to its stabilizing effect on the skin barrier to help retain moisture and the fact that it penetrates quickly; a review published in the *Journal of Cosmetic Dermatology* included EPO among the Top 10 botanical ingredients currently used.

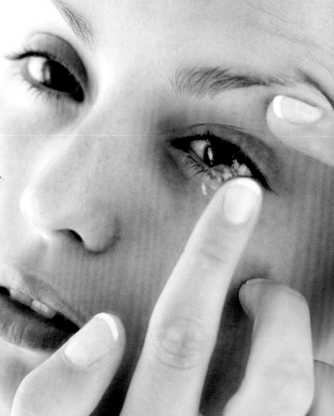

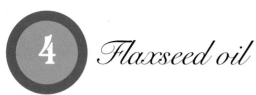

4 *Flaxseed oil*

Especially popular among Ancient Egyptian women, flaxseed oil has been valued as a health and beauty tonic for over 5,000 years. It is one of the richest plant sources of omega-3 essential fatty acids and of oestrogen-like plant hormones known as lignans.

★ *Top tip*

Medicinal flaxseed oil degrades on exposure to light and, if not processed and stored properly, quickly turns rancid. Liquid flaxseed oil must be stored in the refrigerator in an opaque bottle. Avoid oil that is past its use-by date, or which has a strong odour.

On the inside

The omega-3 fatty acids found in flaxseed oil (alpha-linolenic acid) are incorporated into cell membranes to make them more fluid and supple. In the skin, this helps to improve smoothness and elasticity as well as improving the ability to retain moisture and act as an effective barrier against allergens and irritants.

Omega-3s also have a beneficial effect on immune function to increase resistance against infection, and an anti-inflammatory effect that helps to damp down skin breakouts and soothe sensitive skin and inflammatory conditions such as eczema and psoriasis. Research shows that taking flaxseed oil can significantly decrease water loss from the skin by 10 per cent within six weeks, leading to decreased skin sensitivity and improved roughness and scaling within twelve weeks (smoothness and hydration were noticeably increased compared with those taking safflower seed oil, which is low in omega-3s and rich on omega-6s, or placebo).

Flaxseed lignans (found in ground flaxseed rather than the oil) are especially helpful for menopausal women and those with hormone imbalances linked with premenstrual syndrome and painful periods. By interacting with skin oestrogen receptors, they provide a weak hormone-replacement boost to improve collagen and elastin production.

For dry eyes Taking a 1 g or 2 g flaxseed oil capsule per day helps to reduce eye inflammation and feelings of burning and grittiness to improve eye comfort.

Recommended dose Taking flaxseed oil in the form of ground seeds (sprinkled on food) or capsules is the most convenient way to take internally, due to the rapid degradation of oil exposed to light. Flaxseed is always best taken with food to enhance absorption.
- **oil:** 1 tsp to 1 tbsp once or twice a day
- **flaxseeds:** 1–2 tbsp with water twice a day
- **capsules:** 500 mg to 2 g per day

Caution

It is important not to confuse medicinal, cold-pressed flaxseed oil extracted from ripe linseed with the toxic raw linseed oil (from immature seed) used by artists and furniture makers. The latter contains warnings that it should not be taken internally.

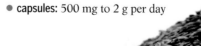

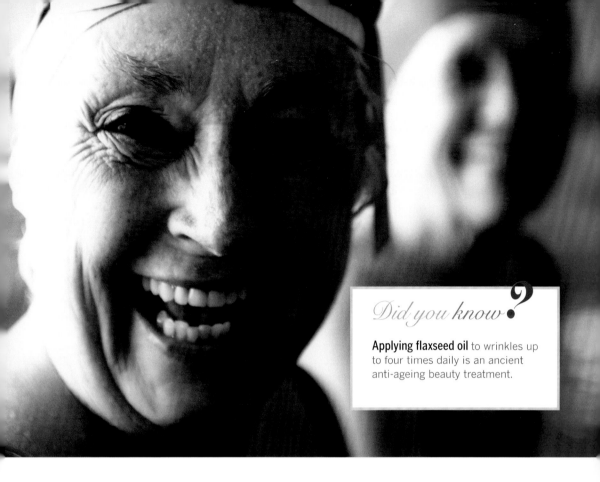

Did you know ?

Applying flaxseed oil to wrinkles up to four times daily is an ancient anti-ageing beauty treatment.

On the outside

Flaxseed oil helps to seal moisture into the skin and it is commonly added to body lotions, sunscreens and dry-skin treatment creams.

Beauty secrets

● Apply neat flaxseed oil to the face and body as a moisturizing, evening treatment to reduce fine lines and wrinkles, and to combat dryness, blemishes and areas of irritation. Use oil from a freshly opened capsule, leave on your face for 15 minutes, then blot off the excess with a tissue and apply your usual night cream. Studies show that, within four months, this can improve skin firmness, elasticity, texture and tone.

● Apply a small amount of oil to your hair to help promote hair growth and lustre, as well as reduce dandruff, scalp-flaking and oil (sebum) production. Regular use makes hair more manageable, soft and shiny, and reduces the static that causes 'fly-away' hair.

● Use warmed flaxseed oil as a deep hair conditioner to lock moisture into the hair and control oil secretion. Alternatively, add a few drops of oil to your hair along with your regular conditioner and rinse well.

5 *Rosehip seed oil*

A rich source of omega-3s, rosehip seed oil also contains tretinoin – a vitamin A derivative used medically to stimulate growth of skin fibroblast cells to plump up and minimize fine lines, wrinkles and acne scars.

On the inside

Rosehip syrup is a rich source of antioxidants, including vitamins C and E plus carotenoids such as lutein, betacarotene and lycopene. Recent research has identified additional, powerful phenolic antioxidants, including anthocyanins, which have an anti-ageing effect on the skin. They are currently being researched for their potential as dietary supplements and for addition to anti-ageing functional foods.

Rosehips also have an antiseptic action; mouthwash made from rosehips has been shown to be effective in reducing the inflammation and pain of recurrent mouth ulcers. They were a popular remedy used by the Ancient Egyptians, Mayans and Native Americans as a tonic, providing vitamin C, vitamin E and substances that have an aspirin-like painkilling action.

Rosehip tea

Simmer 1 tbsp of cut rosehips in 300 ml (1/2 pt) water for 10 minutes to make a medicinal tea.

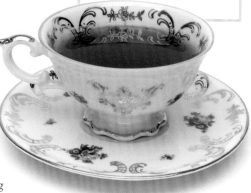

On the outside

Rosehip oil has a light, non-greasy texture and is quickly absorbed into the skin, replenishing moisture and creating a protective barrier to maintain hydration. It is recommended by cosmetic surgeons and included in many skincare products used to treat dermatitis, eczema and acne and to help combat the signs of ageing. Studies have found that applying rosehip seed oil directly to the skin helps to stimulate the growth and rejuvenation of healthy skin cells (keratinocytes).

Reduce scarring Research involving patients with pronounced scars following surgery, injury, burns or radiotherapy showed that Rosa Mosqueta oil reduced redness, thickness and improved suppleness and elasticity, resulting in a significantly improved appearance.

Caution

If you have sensitive, eczema-prone skin, apply a small test amount of oil first, to ensure you don't have an adverse reaction.

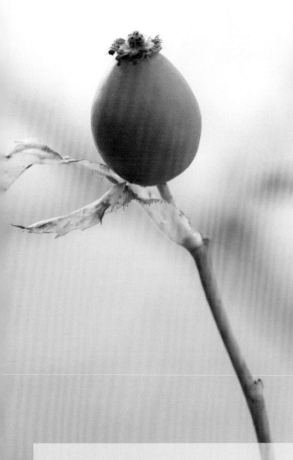

Rosehips improve skin appearance and have an antiseptic action.

Treat damaged or hyperpigmented skin

When applied daily to surface wrinkles, age spots and hyperpigmented areas in women with sun-damaged facial skin, significant improvements were seen after just three weeks. Surface wrinkling reduced, skin became softer and smoother, and brown hyperpigmentation almost completely faded within four months.

Beauty secrets

- **Apply neat to the skin** to moisturize, soften and reduce uneven texture and pigmentation while improving elasticity and providing a radiant glow. Massage in with fingertips until complete absorbed.
- **Apply to spots** to boost healing of blemishes.
- **Apply to scars and burns** to fade redness – even those that are many years old. Rosa Mosqueta oil is also used to treat and prevent the over-formation of scar tissue (raised keloid scars).
- **Apply neat to hair** to strengthen damaged, brittle strands. It can also be rubbed into the scalp to overcome dryness and itching.
- **Apply to nails** to strengthen nail plates and soften cuticles.

QUALITY COUNTS

The best-quality rosehip seed oil comes from an Andean rose, known in Chile as oil of Rosa Mosqueta. Select rosehip seed oil that is cold-pressed rather than solvent-extracted, as this retains the most beneficial nutrients.

6 *Wheatgerm oil*

Wheatgerm oil contains a variety of beneficial fatty acids, including linoleic, oleic and palmitic acids, and is widely used to improve skin dryness, reduce irritation and promote youthful skin.

Wheatgerm oil is cold-pressed from the 'germ' or embryo at the centre of wheat kernels. The germ is the most nutritious part of the kernel and contains numerous vitamins, minerals, proteins and oils. As the germ is such a tiny part of each kernel, however, it takes 18 kg (40 lb) of wheat to produce just one gram of wheatgerm oil. Unfortunately, the wheatgerm is removed during the refining of flour, so it's not present in bread unless replaced later to make an enriched, healthier product.

Wheatgerm oil is a lovely golden amber colour, with a delicious, nutty aroma and flavour. It consists of beneficial monounsaturated and polyunsaturated fats and is among the richest nutritional sources of vitamins E and K. It also provides an abundance of waxy substances such as octacosanol (believed to improve circulation and oxygen delivery to body tissues) and ceramides, which act as signalling molecules to trigger cellular regeneration. In the skin, ceramides form a barrier that prevents excessive water loss and dryness, as well as protecting against UV light and infection.

On the inside

Antioxidant vitamin E obtained from wheatgerm oil has anti-ageing properties that may help to reduce premature fine lines, wrinkles and age spots. It helps to preserve the texture and tone of skin and promotes the growth of healthy hair and nails.

Studies in women with dry skin have found that those who took wheatgerm oil extracts noticed a significant improvement within one to three months, with reduced itching and skin roughness and improved suppleness and hydration on the legs and face.

In your diet Wheatgerm oil is best consumed raw, drizzled over salads, soups, bread, cereal, yogurt or even ice cream.

On the outside

Wheatgerm oil is used to enrich many face creams, shampoos and conditioners, and, although it's thick and sticky, it is readily absorbed into the skin as an effective moisturizer. It has a strong, nutty aroma, so you may prefer to blend it with other cosmetic oils such as argan, coconut, macadamia or rosehip. Some people also like to add a drop or two of lavender essential oil for an enhanced fragrance.

Caution

Do not consume or apply wheatgerm oil if you have a wheat or gluten allergy.

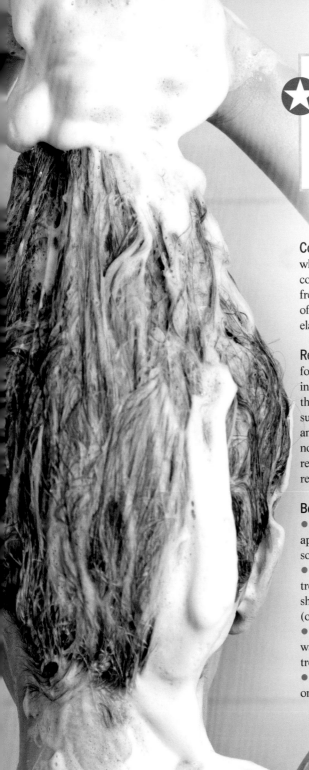

★ *Top tip*

Wheatgerm oil is sensitive to light, so store it in a dark bottle, in the refrigerator, to help keep it fresh.

Combat sagging Research suggests that wheatgerm ceramides help to protect collagen-forming cells in the skin against free-radical damage and reduce the activity of an enzyme, elastase, that breaks down elastin fibres and contributes to sagging.

Regenerate skin Wheatgerm oil is valued for treating dry and mature skin, and is included in anti-ageing products as well as those designed for use on skin conditions such as psoriasis, eczema, stretch marks and scars. It leaves the skin smooth, nourished and hydrated, and promotes regeneration and healing as well as reducing itching.

Beauty secrets

- Rub a few drops between your fingers and apply to hair ends for added gloss and softness.
- Massage a few drops into your scalp to treat dryness and flakiness. Cover with a shower cap and shampoo after 15 minutes (or leave overnight).
- Add a few drops to your shampoo when washing, for a 2-in-1 conditioning treatment.
- Massage a few drops into cracked skin on heels and elbows.

7 *Macadamia nuts*

These delicious nuts consist of 75 per cent fat by weight, of which 80 per cent is beneficial monounsaturated fats. Almost 10 per cent of their weight consists of protein, which, combined with their healthy oil content, makes them especially beneficial for hair, skin and nails.

On the inside

The unique taste and crunch of macadamia nuts hides their high oil content. They have one of the highest levels of beneficial monounsaturated fats found in any food. They are also a good source of magnesium, calcium and vitamins E, B_1, B_2, B_3, B_5, B_6 and folate, all of which are needed by cells with a rapid turnover, such as those in the skin and hair follicles. Macadamias contain numerous antioxidant polyphenols that have anti-inflammatory actions and which improve the ability of blood vessels to dilate to boost blood flow to the skin and scalp.

Eating a handful of macadamia nuts per day has been shown to significantly improve inflammation, making them a good choice

for people with inflammatory skin conditions such as dandruff, rosacea, acne, eczema or psoriasis. They can also help to soothe sunburn, dry skin, dry hair and brittle nails.

In your diet Enjoy a handful of macadamia nuts as a snack, or add them to cereals, desserts, yogurts and salads. The oil is delicious used in salad dressings.

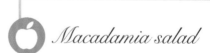

Macadamia salad

For a quick and easy delicious salad, toss together a bag of mixed baby salad leaves, a handful of crushed macadamia nuts and 30 ml (1 fl oz) macadamia nut oil. Serve immediately.

Top tip

When applying macadamia nut oil to your hair, avoid the roots and apply to damaged shafts and hair ends only, to leave hair looking shiny and feeling silky.

On the outside

Macadamia nut oil is included in many shampoos, conditioners and hair masks to help repair damaged hair, nourish hair follicles, smooth roughened hair shafts and extend the life of hair-colouring treatments. When applied to the hair, skin and nails, macadamia oil rapidly sinks in. This deep moisturizing and nourishing action promotes the growth of soft, healthy, voluminous hair that feels and looks thicker. As long as you don't use too much, it will leave hair and skin with a satin sheen rather than an oily residue.

When applied to the skin, macadamia nut oil helps to damp down inflammation and reduce blemishes, even for people with naturally oily skin. It mimics your skin's natural oils, making it an ideal treatment to moisturize dry areas, promote healthy cell membranes and support skin-healing.

Beauty secrets

- Apply a small amount of neat oil to tame unruly hair as well as reduce drying time after washing.
- Use as a body oil to moisturize skin after a bath or shower.
- Use a little oil as a make-up remover to cleanse the skin and gently melt away even the most stubborn mascara. As an additional benefit, it acts like a serum to sink in and nourish delicate skin around the eyes.

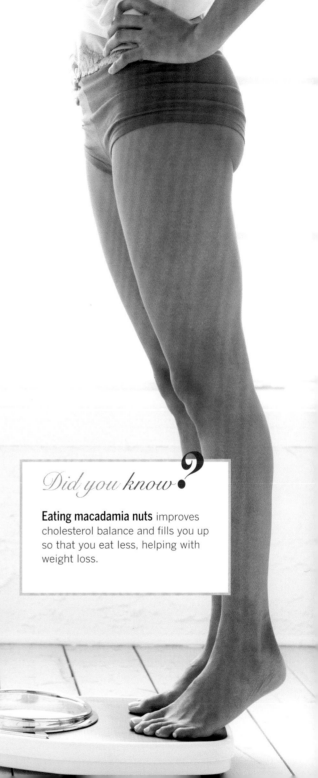

Did you know?

Eating macadamia nuts improves cholesterol balance and fills you up so that you eat less, helping with weight loss.

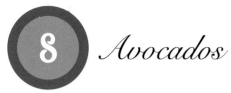

Avocados

Avocados are a rich source of healthy, monounsaturated fatty acids. They also provide one of the highest protein contents of any fruit, plus B vitamins, antioxidant vitamins C and E, antioxidant carotenoid pigments and magnesium.

Though rich in monounsaturated fats, these are incorporated into a water-based matrix that masks any oiliness. Unlike most fruits, avocados only start to ripen and fulfil their nutritional potential once cut from the tree. They should be stored at room temperature until the flesh softens sufficiently to use.

Avocado oil has a rich, green colour. Only select cold-pressed oils, not the cheaper, refined versions which contain less of the active ingredients.

On the inside

Avocado oil contains hormone-like phytosterols that have a regenerative effect on ageing skin. While you can use it during cooking, it's best to drizzle cold-pressed avocado oil over salads and dips to retain the full benefits and to enhance the absorption of other ingredients. Just adding chopped avocado or avocado oil to salsa, for example, enhances the absorption of beneficial tomato pigments (lycopene and betacarotene) fourfold, compared with avocado-free salsa.

Soothe inflammatory skin conditions

Avocado oil is a useful treatment for dry, inflammatory skin conditions such as acne, dermatitis, eczema, psoriasis and rosacea. When consumed, its healthy fats are converted into anti-inflammatory substances that help to damp down redness and inflammation. When applied as a cream containing vitamin B_{12} and avocado oil, psoriasis plaques have been found to improve significantly.

Protect against premature ageing

Several studies suggest that the antioxidant pigments found in avocados (especially lutein and zeaxanthin) help to protect DNA against premature ageing. Studies have shown that airline pilots and frequent air travellers with high intakes of these nutrients showed significantly less DNA damage than those with low intakes, suggesting that these substances have an anti-ageing effect. Skin shows the first visible signs of ageing, and avocado pigments appear to protect against UV damage. In addition, researchers have found that avocado extracts also help to protect skin by enhancing wound-healing.

In your diet Avocado makes a great starter, served with a dash of vinaigrette or mixed with prawns and a light cocktail sauce.

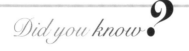

Did you know?

Dietary surveys show that people who regularly consume avocados have higher levels of 'good' HDL-cholesterol, lower blood pressure, better glucose control, plus a lower weight and waist circumference than non-consumers.

Or mash with olive oil and garlic to make guacamole, serve sliced with tomatoes and mozzarella cheese for a tricolour salad, or cook in a vegetable, avocado and cheese bake. Be creative!

On the outside

Avocado oil is an increasingly popular beauty treatment that, according to some, is more hydrating and penetrates more deeply than coconut oil. Try using it on a cotton-wool pad to remove make-up, then massage in the residue as a moisturizing night serum. A little goes a long way, as it takes 10–15 minutes for full absorption.

Or why not use fresh avocado to give yourself a facial? It can be used for all skin types, as outlined in these beauty tips:

Beauty secrets
● **Use chilled avocado peel** (save the peel when using avocado in the kitchen) to gently rub over your face to absorb the healthy oils.
● **Place a thin avocado slice** under each eye to reduce puffiness.
● **Make a simple mask for dry skin** by mashing a ripe avocado, and apply to the face. Lie back and relax for 15 minutes, then rinse. Use any leftovers to massage into your hands and feet – especially cracked heels.
● **Make a mask for oily skin** by combining the mashed flesh of a small, ripe avocado with one egg white, 1 tbsp of rolled oats and 1 tbsp of lemon juice. Leave on for 20 minutes, then rinse.

Avocados contain mannoheptulose – a sugar that helps satisfy sensations of hunger.

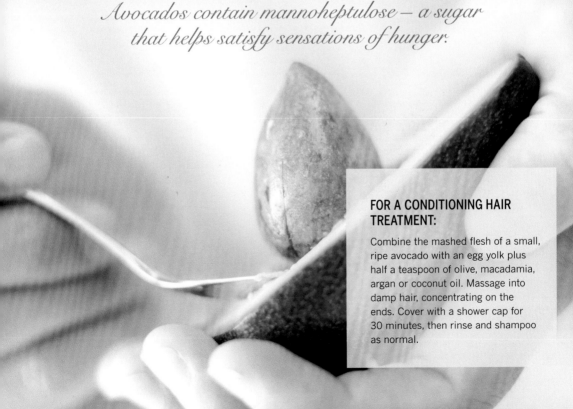

FOR A CONDITIONING HAIR TREATMENT:

Combine the mashed flesh of a small, ripe avocado with an egg yolk plus half a teaspoon of olive, macadamia, argan or coconut oil. Massage into damp hair, concentrating on the ends. Cover with a shower cap for 30 minutes, then rinse and shampoo as normal.

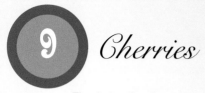

Cherries

The darker the cherry, the more benefits it offers. The dark pigments are anthocyanins with a powerful antioxidant action, so black cherry juice – along with tart, dark-red cherries – provides the highest antioxidant potency of just about any fruit or vegetable.

The antioxidants found in cherries protect their skins from wrinkling in strong sunlight and, when consumed, they provide similar protection against premature ageing for human skin, too.

Researchers have recently found that cherries (especially the tart Balaton and Montmorency strains) contain five times more melatonin than other fruit sources such as blackberries and strawberries. In fruit, melatonin contributes to the antioxidant protection against sun exposure and also has beneficial effects on root growth. In humans, melatonin acts as a hormone in the brain that helps to regulate the sleep–wake cycle. As well as ensuring you obtain sufficient beauty sleep, melatonin boosts immunity and is also produced in your skin, where it protects against the harmful, ageing effects of ultraviolet light.

All cherries are also a good source of vitamin C – vital for promoting collagen production in skin.

On the inside

Skin cells exposed to ultraviolet light are twice as likely to survive when melatonin levels are high. Scientists from Michigan State University have suggested that drinking a glass of red cherry juice a day can help to slow the ageing process. Consuming cherries brings other benefits, too:

Combat wrinkles Researchers assessing the food intake of over 400 people aged over seventy, living in Greece, Australia and Sweden, discovered that cherries are one of the fruits that offer most protection against skin wrinkling, with those having the highest

Did you know?

Tart or sour cherries, which are used in baking, provide twice as many anti-ageing antioxidants as sweet cherries. However, eating sweet cherries every day can reduce your blood levels of inflammatory chemicals by up to 20 per cent.

intakes experiencing 46 per cent fewer signs of skin ageing.

Get a good night's sleep Research from Louisiana State University suggests that drinking Montmorency cherry juice, twice a day for two weeks, increases sleep time in people with insomnia. Those drinking the cherry juice slept for more than an hour longer each night (averaging 84 minutes), compared with those drinking a placebo juice. Red cherry pigments (proanthocyanidins) also play a role by increasing the availability of tryptophan, an essential amino acid needed to produce melatonin in the body.

Alleviate inflammatory conditions
By reducing inflammation, eating cherries and drinking cherry juice helps to damp down the redness of acne, eczema, psoriasis, rosacea and other skin rashes.

On the outside

Cherries are included in many products designed to fade dark spots and help lighten skin tone. Some researchers believe they also have regenerative and rejuvenating skin properties, thanks to their unusually high level of antioxidants.

Beauty secrets
● Make a simple, anti-ageing skin mask by removing the stones from ripe cherries and mashing the flesh with a garlic press. Apply to your face for 15 minutes, then rinse.
● Make a mask for dry skin by adding a few drops of your favourite oil – evening primrose, coconut or rosehip – plus a teaspoon of honey to the mask above.

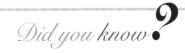

Did you know?

Despite tasting sharp, tart or sour, cherries have an alkaline effect in the body to help maintain an ideal pH balance in your skin.

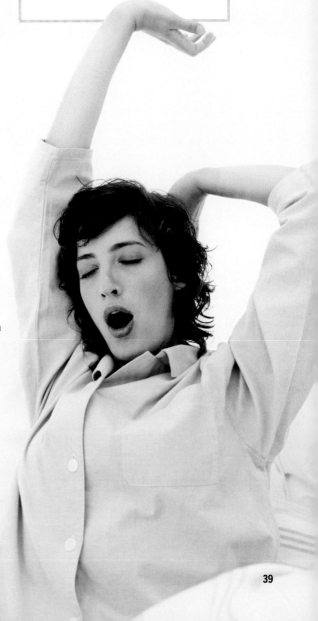

10 *Bilberries*

Also known as wild blueberries and blue whortleberries, bilberries contain a richer blend of antioxidant pigments called anthocyanins. Like other berries, they are also rich in vitamin C.

Bilberry extracts strengthen blood vessels by stimulating the production of collagen. They also have a diuretic action and are used medicinally to reduce fluid retention, easy bruising, thread veins and eye problems affecting blood vessels in the retina. Their antioxidant action is also believed to protect against cataracts.

Although not always easy to find fresh out of season, some stores stock them frozen or bottled – and you can always grow your own! Capsules are also widely available.

On the inside

Bilberry antioxidants are great for the skin, and help to reduce premature ageing, soothe inflammatory conditions such as acne, and improve the appearance of cellulite. A regular intake of bilberries is said to improve skin plumpness and glow, partly due to the presence of anti-ageing resveratrol and quercetin.

Alleviate skin conditions Bilberry has been utilized as a cure for numerous skin conditions, such as skin ulcers and varicose veins. As frequent ingestion of bilberry assists in enhancing blood circulation, it has also been used to fight venous deficit, which in turn causes certain skin difficulties.

Boost circulation Bilberry extracts are used to increase circulation, reduce fluid retention and, if you have varicose veins, can improve feelings of leg heaviness and pins and needles, as well as improving the appearance of overlying skin.

Improve eye health Bilberry pigments help to stabilize tear production, increase blood flow to the retina and regenerate the light-sensitive pigment rhodopsin. Some researchers have even found that taking bilberry extracts can reduce short-sightedness after five months of regular use, through an effect on the eye lens. Bilberry extracts are therefore a popular choice to reduce puffiness and dark circles, and to promote bright, healthy eyes.

Recommended dose If taking as a supplement, take 80–160 mg, one to three times a day.

In your diet Like the closely related blueberry (which has a creamy-coloured flesh and lower antioxidant content), bilberries can be included in jams and muffins, and dolloped on cereals, pancakes, yogurt and even ice cream.

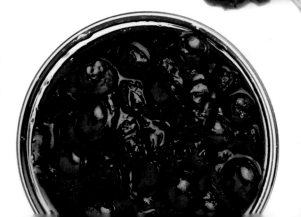

Did you know?

British World War II pilots ate bilberry jam to help improve their night vision.

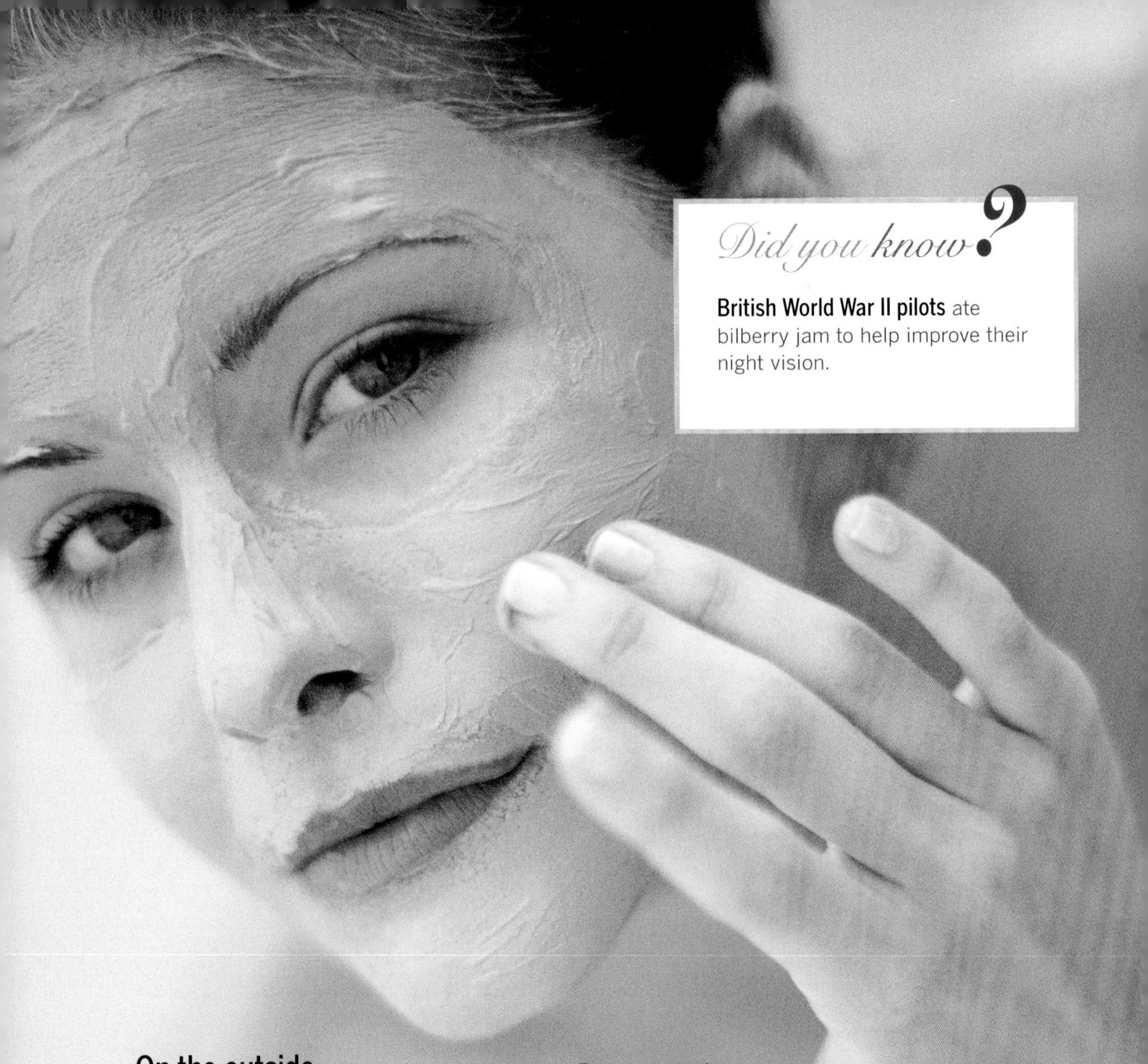

On the outside

Bilberry extracts are often included in anti-ageing creams, face masks and sun lotions. In laboratory tests, they have been found to reduce skin cell damage on exposure to UVA and UVB light. Researchers are now working to improve the antioxidant activity of blueberry-containing creams by enclosing them in nano-sized 'liposomes' to penetrate the skin more deeply.

Beauty secrets

- **Make a bilberry mask** to lighten pigmentation and discourage blemishes:
  - **For oily skin:** simply blend a handful of fresh/defrosted bilberries to form a paste. Apply to skin for 20 minutes, then rinse.
  - **For dry skin:** add a tablespoon of fresh yogurt and a teaspoon of macadamia, rosehip, wheatgerm or avocado oils to the bilberries; blend, and use as above.

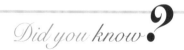

11 *Acai berries*

These small, purple-black berries have a long history of use to help the skin look younger and fresher, and also for treating inflammatory skin conditions such as acne and rosacea.

Acai berries are obtained from a Brazilian palm tree, *Euterpe oleracea*. Outside of South America, they are mainly available as powder or tablet supplements prepared by flash freezing. The level of antioxidants found in fresh acai juice, which includes vitamin C and flavonoids, is similar to that of cranberries, and greater than orange or apple juice. Freeze-dried acai powder, however, has one of the highest antioxidant levels of any food tested, and can double or even triple the level of antioxidant protection normally found in the circulation.

Did you know?

Acai has a similar anti-inflammatory, painkilling action as aspirin, though the effect is weaker.

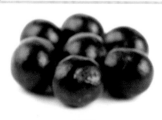

On the inside

Acai berries are high in healthy omega fats and also contain valuable phytosterols and anthocyanins, with a greater antioxidant capacity than any other berry. They are a good source of calcium, iron, magnesium and zinc, and are an unusually rich source of the trace element manganese, which is important for maintaining healthy skin, nails, hair and hair colour. The presence of oestrogen-like plant hormones, known as lignans, helps to boost collagen and elastin production in the skin and may reduce the appearance of fine lines and wrinkles.

The ripe berries have an exotic flavour and, in South America, are used to make smoothies, juices, jam and ice cream. Acai juice is said to help flush excess water from the body to reduce puffiness and dark circles around the eyes.

Recommended dose Acai supplements are usually taken at a dose of between 500 mg and 1 g concentrated extracts daily.

On the outside

When cold pressed, acai seeds yield a green oil which is highly antioxidant and rich in both monounsaturated and omega-3 essential fatty acids. The oil can be applied to the skin as an antioxidant, anti-ageing protectant.

Beauty secrets

If visiting Brazil, apply fresh acai pulp as an indulgent, antioxidant face mask. If using oil:
● **Apply acai oil topically** to treat patchy skin colouring (hyperpigmentation caused by excess melanin production).
● **Apply a small amount of oil** to hair that is dry or damaged, especially from colouring.

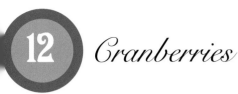

12 *Cranberries*

Cranberries are well-known for their ability to protect against urinary tract infections, but this antimicrobial action also protects against the formation of dental plaque, tooth decay, receding gums and bad breath.

On the inside

Cranberries are a good source of vitamins (B$_1$, B$_2$, B$_3$, B$_5$, B$_6$, C, E, K) and minerals (including calcium, iron, magnesium, manganese and zinc), all of which are important for skin and circulation, helping to maintain a healthy glow. They also provide a broad range of complexion-boosting antioxidants, including a unique type of proanthocyanidin that is responsible for their antimicrobial effects.

Detox your skin Cranberry juice is often recommended to detoxify the skin, especially if you are prone to acne or dry, scaly skin – or the opposite problem of oily skin.

Recommended dose If taking cranberry fruit extracts, the usual dose is 500 mg daily.

In your diet These sour red fruits are most commonly used to make sauces and jellies, or enjoyed as a refreshing fruit drink, but why not try baking with them (in both savoury and sweet dishes) or using them to make a quick salsa, too?

On the outside

Cranberry oil is added to many anti-ageing products, as its antioxidants help to reduce

Did you know?

Cranberry juice naturally has a similar level of sugar and acidity as lemon juice. To make an acceptable drink, the juice is diluted to around 27 per cent juice concentration, and sweetened to around the same level as apple or grape juice. Low-sugar versions made with artificial sweeteners are available, too. Recommended juice intakes are 200–300 ml (7–10 fl oz) daily.

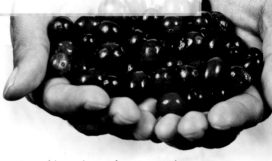

premature skin ageing and protect against fine lines and wrinkles. It is easily absorbed to moisturize the skin, improving hydration, elasticity, texture and brightening the complexion. Cranberry oil is also soothing, helping to reduce skin inflammation, redness, itchiness and other signs of irritation.

Beauty secrets
● Make an exfoliating, antibacterial face mask by mixing together unsweetened cranberry juice (or crushed pulp), oatmeal, manuka honey and olive oil. Leave on for 5 minutes, then gently rub into skin to exfoliate and wash off.
● Enhance colour and shine of red-brown hair and reduce dandruff by rinsing your hair with diluted, unsweetened cranberry juice (dilute 1:1 with water) straight after washing.

13 Blackberries, strawberries & raspberries

Berries are among the most beneficial of fruits. They contain relatively little sugar compared to other fruit and are low in calories, typically supplying only 25 kcal per 100 g (3½ oz). They're packed full of minerals, vitamin C and antioxidants, too.

The unique anti-ageing antioxidants that berries contain protect them from sunlight, as well as contributing to their delicious aroma, taste and colour. Those that are dark red, purple or black have the highest antioxidant content; if you ever find black raspberries on sale, or growing wild, snap them up for their particularly high content of dark purple anthocyanins. Berry seeds are also rich in omega-3s and beneficial omega-6 fatty acids, which are essential for healthy skin.

Did you know?

Strawberries are one of the few natural fruit sources of iodine, lack of which is associated with a slow metabolism, coarse skin, and brittle hair and nails.

On the inside

The vitamin C provided by eating berries is vital for collagen production in the skin. People with higher vitamin C intakes have fewer wrinkles and less dry skin. Substances such as ellagic acid, which protect berries from sunlight, have a similar effect on the skin to reduce sunburn and sun damage. Researchers conducting studies comparing dietary intakes with degree of skin wrinkling found that those with good intakes of fruit salads containing strawberries/berries showed 36 per cent fewer signs of skin ageing than those with low intakes.

In your diet Enjoy berries on their own, add to cereals, yogurt, fruit salad or desserts, or whizz them up into delicious smoothies.

On the outside

Strawberries are widely used in skincare products, as they contain alpha-hydroxy fruit acids with a gentle bleaching action, to refresh and soften the skin for a gentle glow. Raspberries are used for their astringency, helping to tighten pores, as well as their softening and anti-ageing effects, while blackberries are both hydrating and anti-ageing.

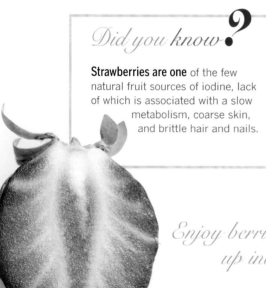

Enjoy berries on their own, or whizz them up into delicious smoothies …

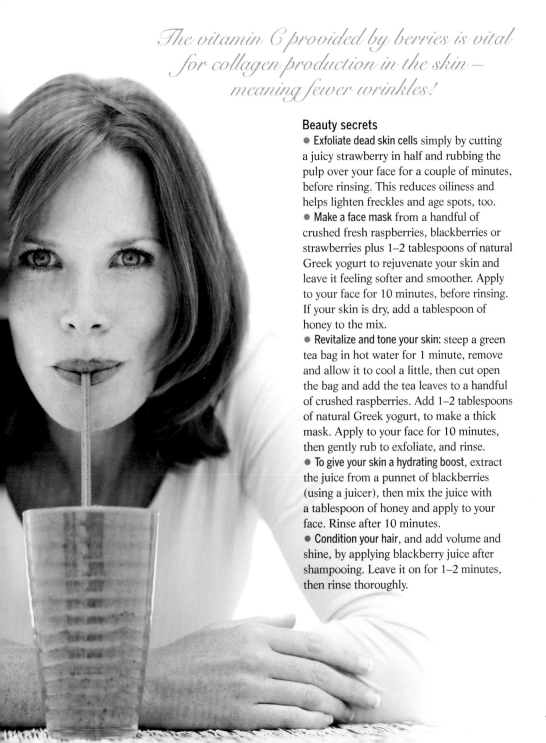

The vitamin C provided by berries is vital for collagen production in the skin — meaning fewer wrinkles!

Beauty secrets

- **Exfoliate dead skin cells** simply by cutting a juicy strawberry in half and rubbing the pulp over your face for a couple of minutes, before rinsing. This reduces oiliness and helps lighten freckles and age spots, too.
- **Make a face mask** from a handful of crushed fresh raspberries, blackberries or strawberries plus 1–2 tablespoons of natural Greek yogurt to rejuvenate your skin and leave it feeling softer and smoother. Apply to your face for 10 minutes, before rinsing. If your skin is dry, add a tablespoon of honey to the mix.
- **Revitalize and tone your skin:** steep a green tea bag in hot water for 1 minute, remove and allow it to cool a little, then cut open the bag and add the tea leaves to a handful of crushed raspberries. Add 1–2 tablespoons of natural Greek yogurt, to make a thick mask. Apply to your face for 10 minutes, then gently rub to exfoliate, and rinse.
- **To give your skin a hydrating boost,** extract the juice from a punnet of blackberries (using a juicer), then mix the juice with a tablespoon of honey and apply to your face. Rinse after 10 minutes.
- **Condition your hair,** and add volume and shine, by applying blackberry juice after shampooing. Leave it on for 1–2 minutes, then rinse thoroughly.

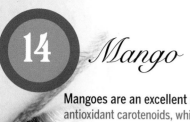

14 *Mango*

Mangoes are an excellent source of antioxidant carotenoids, which help to protect your skin against the harmful, ageing effects of sunlight, with some varieties containing as much as 3 g carotenoid pigments per 100 g (3½ oz) flesh.

Certain carotenoids, such as betacarotene, can be converted in the body to vitamin A (retinol) when needed. Vitamin A – as well as being an antioxidant itself – has a direct effect of switching on genes needed for the synthesis of proteins, and is important for collagen production in healthy skin.

Did you know?

Vitamin A derivatives are used medically to treat acne, psoriasis and sun damage (photo-ageing), including wrinkles.

Top tip

The best way to eat a fresh mango is to slice it lengthways into thirds, discard the centre third containing the stone, and to score the flesh of the two outer thirds into a criss-cross pattern. Turn these outer sections inside out, so the flesh is presented in bite-sized cubes that are easy to remove from the peel.

On the inside

Mangoes are such a rich source of carotenoids that they help to prevent lack of vitamin A; lack of this vitamin can lead to rough, scaly skin with raised, pimply hair follicles – a condition known as keratosis pilaris – plus flaky scalp and dull, brittle hair. They are also a rich source of vitamin C, which is also needed for collagen synthesis. Women over the age of forty who have higher intakes of vitamin C have been shown to have fewer skin wrinkles and less dryness than those with low intakes.

On the outside

Mango is added to numerous skin and hair products with a tropical aroma. It's also a great way to combat blackheads (see below).

Beauty secrets
● **To treat blackheads,** mix a teaspoon of mango pulp with a teaspoon of manuka honey and rub over your face using a circular motion. Leave on for 10–20 minutes, then rinse. As well as exfoliating skin and blackheads, it will add a healthy glow.

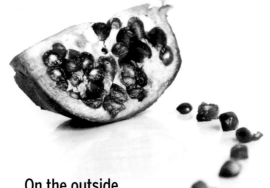

15 _Pomegranate_

The ruby juice of the pomegranate is exceptionally rich in antioxidants, including vitamin C, red carotenoid pigments and polyphenols such as catechins and ellagic acid, which help protect the skin against sun damage.

On the inside

Ultraviolet radiation from the sun is one of the main causes of premature skin ageing. Drinking pomegranate juice helps to protect your skin against sun damage by suppressing the oxidation of skin cells' membranes (a process known as lipid peroxidation) and boosting your skin's natural sun protection factor by around one quarter. It is also said to improve hair growth and lustre.

In addition, pomegranate fruit extracts have been found to have a beneficial effect in the mouth, inhibiting the bacteria that cause dental plaque, bad breath and tooth decay.

In your diet Drinking 250 ml (¹/₂ pt) of pomegranate juice significantly improves the antioxidant level of blood and provides similar antioxidant activity to green tea. You can also throw the seeds into salads and rice dishes, for a Middle Eastern twist.

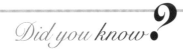

Pomegranate oil is beneficial even for oily skin, as it helps to combat breakouts, reduce scarring and soothe irritation.

On the outside

Pomegranate extracts from the fruit, peel and seeds are widely included in skin creams and serums, penetrating deeply to reduce fine lines and wrinkles and repair sun damage. Pomegranate seed oil stimulates the division of epidermal skin cells, promoting smooth, firm skin, while pomegranate peel extracts stimulate the production of collagen in the dermis and suppresses the enzymes that break it down. These actions help to replenish dry, dull, thinning skin and reverse some of the visible signs of ageing.

Pomegranate supports the healing of blemishes and improves sun protection factor (SPF) by around 20 per cent. It also has a natural lightening and brightening action to combat a dull or mottled complexion, staining and freckles (pomegranate fruit extracts directly inhibit the gene responsible for producing tyrosinase, an enzyme involved in melanin synthesis in skin cells). The seed extracts have an antimicrobial action to reduce skin blemishes, too.

Beauty secrets

● **Tame dry, frizzy hair** by applying warm pomegranate seed oil as an intensive-care treatment. Leave on for an hour, then wash as normal.
● **Add shine and softness** to hair by applying a few drops of pomegranate seed oil (warm the oil in your hands first) to dry ends.

16 $\mathcal{P}$apaya

The orange-red flesh of this delicious tropical tree fruit is packed full of lycopene, an antioxidant carotenoid pigment that protects the fruit – and, in turn, our skin – from sun exposure. It also contains vitamin C, B vitamins and minerals such as calcium and magnesium.

On the inside

Papaya (also known as pawpaw) is perhaps best known as a source of papain, a protease enzyme that breaks down protein to aid its digestion and absorption. As you get older, your ability to digest protein may reduce due to falling levels of stomach acids and intestinal enzymes. This can lead to bloating, wind and heartburn. Taking a digestive enzyme supplement containing papain can improve protein digestion and ensure a steady supply of protein building blocks (amino acids) to hair follicles to help reduce hair-thinning.

The lycopene present in raw papaya is up to six times more readily absorbed into the body than the lycopene in raw tomatoes, ensuring maximum protection for the skin.

On the outside

Papaya pulp is included in many facial creams and shampoos, as its alpha-hydroxy fruit acids and papain enzyme help have an anti-ageing effect, brightening skin tone, gently bleaching age spots and 'dissolving' away dead skin cells.

Beauty secrets

● **Rub the peel into your skin** (save the peel when eating fresh papaya) to achieve a healthy glow. Leave on for no more than 5 minutes, then rinse.

● **Make a simple mask** by mashing fresh, ripe papaya, and apply to the face to discourage blemishes, age spots and wrinkles. Rinse after 15 minutes.

● **To hydrate dry skin**, mash half a papaya with a little honey, for a more nourishing mask. You can also add your favourite beauty oil – avocado, evening primrose, coconut or rosehip oil. Rinse after 15 minutes.

● **Make a body scrub** for use in the shower by mashing together ripe papaya pulp with salt and olive oil, to soften and exfoliate skin.

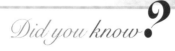
Did you know?

Papaya seeds taste like peppercorns and can be dried and put in a peppermill to make a healthy, spicy seasoning.

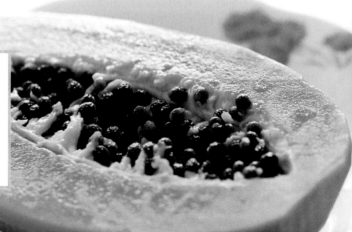

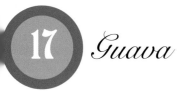

Guava

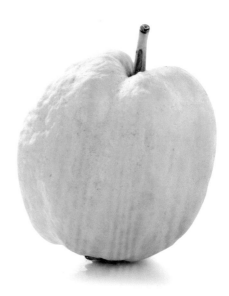

Guavas have a distinctive, lemony aroma. The pulp of this tropical fruit varies in colour from cream to deep pink; those with the darkest colour offer the most benefits. The seeds are also pressed to extract a rich oil.

On the inside

The guava's pink colour is due to the carotenoid pigment lycopene. The lycopene and vitamin C present in guava (and papaya) help to protect your skin against sun damage; lycopene has been shown to reduce the adverse skin-ageing effects of ultraviolet light. High vitamin C intake has also been linked to fewer wrinkles and less skin dryness in middle-aged women.

Drinking guava juice is a popular Asian remedy for acne, pimples and wrinkles.

In your diet Guava may be eaten raw or cooked, and is delicious in Asian sauces and sweet-and-sour dishes. In the West, the juice is more widely available than the fruit.

On the outside

Guava seed oil is widely used in skincare products for its moisture-retention and antioxidant properties. It assists in maintaining skin elasticity, tones and brightens the skin, and helps to prevent premature wrinkles. The oil may also be applied to the scalp to prevent and treat dandruff, reduce hair loss and revitalize hair by restoring shine.

Beauty secrets

If you can get hold of fresh guava, try the following:
- **To treat blackheads, heal blemishes and fade age spots,** crush guava leaves to make a paste. Apply to troublespots, leave for 10 minutes, then rinse.
- **To make a face mask,** cut a guava in half, remove the seeds and place the flesh in a blender together with a tablespoon of ground oatmeal. Whizz together to form a thick paste. Apply to your skin for 10 minutes to tighten pores, reduce oiliness and discourage wrinkles.
- **For an extra-strength mask,** blend two or three tender guava leaves along with the fruit and oatmeal, as above. This enhances the astringent quality of the mask to help heal pimples and dim spots.

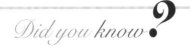

Did you know?

Guavas are the richest fruit source of vitamin C, providing as much as 230 mg per 100 g (3½ oz) of fruit.

Pink grapefruit

Red and pink grapefruit gain their colour from lycopene, the same carotenoid pigment that gives tomatoes, guava, papaya and watermelon their distinctive hues. As grapefruit also provide vitamin C and large amounts of bioactive polyphenols, they offer significant anti-ageing benefits.

Caution

Grapefruit contains substances (such as naringin) that interact with enzymes needed to process some prescribed drugs. If you are on medication, check the drug-information leaflet in case interactions indicate you should not consume grapefruit in any form.

Lycopene is a powerful antioxidant that helps to protect against the ageing effects of free-radical damage (free radicals are molecular fragments that carry a minute, negative electrical charge and cause oxidation reactions). It is three times more potent than vitamin E, and consuming a single lycopene-rich fruit can reduce the oxidative damage to your DNA by as much as 50 per cent within 24 hours.

On the inside

Our skin is at high risk of free-radical damage when exposed to ultraviolet light. This is the main cause of premature skin ageing, yet we also need some sunlight exposure to synthesize vitamin D. Just as lycopene protects tomatoes from sun exposure, eating lycopene-rich fruits, such as red and pink grapefruit, offers some protection.

On the outside

Grapefruit essential oil, extracted from the peel, consists mainly of a powerful antioxidant called limonene. Limonene is added to many perfumes, creams and hair treatments to provide a fresh, citrus aroma and reduce oiliness.

Grapefruit essential oil should not be used neat on the skin, but, like most oils, should be well diluted. Some people are sensitive to the oil, leading to contact dermatitis, so patch-test a small area first.

Beauty secrets

Grapefruit juice is a popular astringent toner, helping to tighten pores and brighten the complexion while combating free radicals:

● **Make a revitalizing mask** by mixing together the juice from half a pink or red grapefruit with 1 tablespoon honey and enough oatmeal to make a thick paste. Apply to your face for 10 minutes, then rinse.

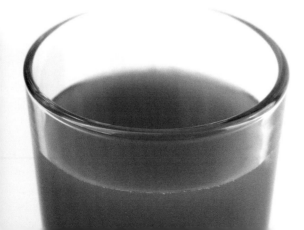

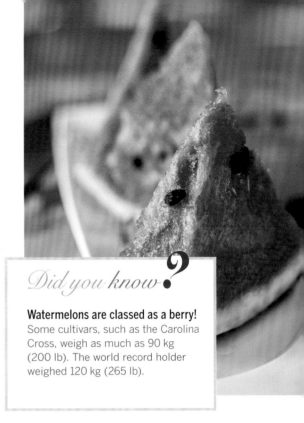

19 *Watermelon*

This distinctive fruit, with its green, mottled or striped rind and deep red flesh dotted with glistening seeds, is a rich source of the carotenoid pigment lycopene, which, together with its vitamin C content, provides anti-ageing benefits for your skin and hair.

While orange-, yellow- and even white-flesh varieties are also available, as are seedless ones, it is the red ones that provide the most protection.

On the inside

Watermelon peel is edible and resembles cucumber in flavour. It is a rich source of an amino acid called citrulline, which is converted into arginine in the body. Arginine has a powerful blood-vessel-dilating action, improving blood flow to the peripheries such as the scalp and nail beds. It is a traditional remedy used to promote hair growth, and to improve sexual function in men and sex drive in women.

Research carried out in Greece, Australia and Sweden on the food intake of more than 400 people aged seventy or over found that melons are one of the fruits that offer the most protection against skin wrinkling; those with the highest intakes experienced 44 per cent fewer signs of skin ageing.

On the outside

Watermelon can be used to tone your skin, tightening pores and reducing oiliness (see following tips).

Did you know?

Watermelons are classed as a berry!
Some cultivars, such as the Carolina Cross, weigh as much as 90 kg (200 lb). The world record holder weighed 120 kg (265 lb).

Beauty secrets

● **Massage the peel into your skin** (if you don't want to eat it), paying special attention to the forehead, nose and chin, which can be prone to oiliness.

● **To treat oily skin**, soak a cotton-wool ball in watermelon juice and apply to clean skin. Leave for 15 minutes before rinsing. If your skin is dry, add a teaspoon of honey to the juice and mix well before using.

● **To soften and gently exfoliate skin**, mix 1 tablespoon of watermelon juice with 1 tablespoon plain Greek yogurt and apply to skin. Leave for 10 minutes before rinsing.

● **For an anti-ageing mask**, mix 1 tablespoon of watermelon juice with 1 tablespoon of mashed avocado and apply to skin. Leave for 20 minutes, then rinse.

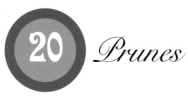

20 Prunes

Despite their brown, wrinkled appearance, prunes offer great anti-ageing potential for your skin. The fact that they contain concentrated dark plum pigments mean they have one of the highest anti-ageing, antioxidant levels of all fruit.

Prunes are made by drying several different varieties of plum, of which the most popular is the d'Agen sugar plum. They are an excellent source of fibre, to help reduce bloating and fluid retention, and a good vegetarian source of iron – needed for the transport of oxygen to actively divide cells that produce hair, skin and nails.

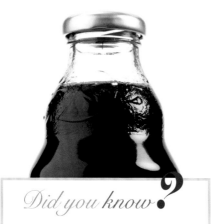

Did you know?

Prune juice has a laxative action, yet only contains a trace of fibre. Its effectiveness is due to the presence of substances (hydroxyphenylisatin) which stimulate secretion of fluid and intestinal contraction.

GET PASTED

In Japan, prune paste is eaten as a delicacy to enhance skin and hair. It is also applied as an anti-ageing mask. If you can get hold of some, why not discover its benefits for yourself – or try the treatment tips recommended opposite (see *Beauty secrets*).

On the inside

Researchers have found that prunes offer unusually high anti-ageing protection against sun damage and skin wrinkling: of those taking part in an international study, people with a high intake of dried prunes showed 42 per cent fewer signs of skin ageing than those with low intakes.

Prune juice is a popular home remedy for reducing acne and pimples, due to its colon-cleansing action. It also supplies vitamins and minerals that nourish hair growth.

In your diet Due to the form of iron they contain, prunes are best eaten with an additional vitamin C source, such as orange juice, to maximize iron absorption.

On the outside

Whether using whole prunes, prune extract (widely available from health-food stores) or prune juice, this dried fruit will soon become a regular part of your beauty regime, once you discover its wide-ranging benefits …

Beauty secrets

- **Make a home-made mask** that's suitable for both dry and oily skin by combining 1 tablespoon of prune extract with 2 tablespoons natural bio yogurt and 1 tablespoon of oats or bran. Leave on for 15 minutes, then rinse off with a gentle exfoliating action.
- **To treat blemish-prone skin**, soak two stone-free prunes overnight in green tea until soft. Drain and mash the prunes, and add 1 tablespoon of oatmeal and 1 tablespoon of manuka honey. Apply to skin, leave on for 20 minutes, then rinse.
- **Enhance hair colour** with prune juice: shampoo and rinse hair as usual, then lean over a bowl or sink and apply prune juice to hair. Scoop up the juice and reapply several times. Cover with a shower cap for 15 minutes, then rinse thoroughly.

Prune juice has a rich, dark amber colour that is used as an alternative to henna to enhance hair colour in some cultures, and to cover a touch of grey.

Age-busting breakfast

Prunes soaked overnight in green tea make a great, anti-ageing breakfast. Sprinkle them with ground flaxseed, dried cranberries and a few shavings of dark chocolate for additional tasty benefits.

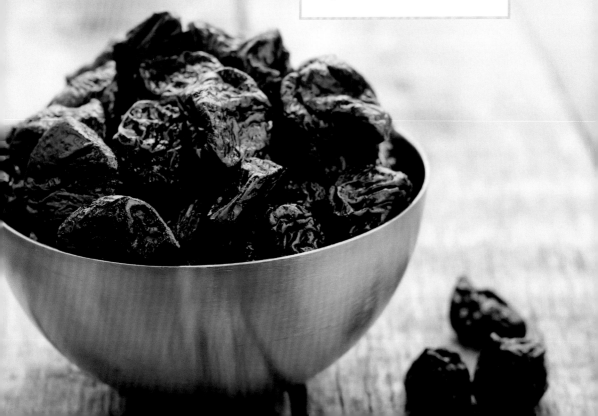

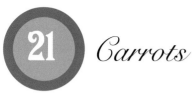

21 Carrots

Carrots contain carotenoids, which help to protect skin cells from premature wrinkles, pigmentation and uneven skin tone. They also contain vitamin C and boost levels of vitamin A, both of which have skin-friendly effects in the body.

Carotenoids are the yellow-orange pigments that give carrots their vibrant colour. As well as having an antioxidant action, to damp down inflammation, these carotenoids – including alpha-carotene and betacarotene – act as pro-vitamins, as they can be converted to vitamin A in the body. Vitamin A, in turn, is used to make rhodopsin, also known as visual purple – a pigment needed for normal vision. Improved vision helps to reduce the squinting and straining that can deepen the fine lines around your eyes.

On the inside

Scientists from St Andrews and Bristol universities in the UK have found that people who eat the most carrots are also considered more attractive. Carotenoids become concentrated in the skin to impart a yellow glow – similar to a suntan – that is interpreted as attractive and healthy, with visible results after just two months of increased consumption. The increased colour also acts as a natural sunblock and can provide some dietary protection against sunburn: a study in the *American Journal of Clinical Nutrition* found that supplementing with 25 mg of carotenoids

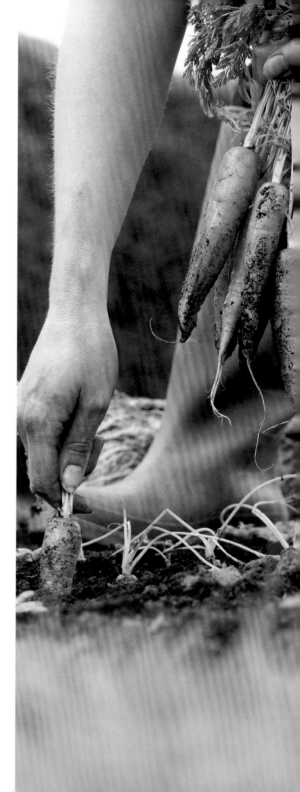

for eight weeks provided significant protection against sunburn. (NOTE: you should still use skin protection if you are planning to spend more than 15 minutes in the sun.)

Research has shown that eating carrots can nurture skin, hair and nail growth, as vitamin A is essential for replenishing cells with a rapid turnover. The antioxidants and carotenoids contained in carrots protect and condition the skin; carrots also contain vitamin C, which is needed for collagen production to maintain skin elasticity.

In your diet Carrots are very low in calories and contain virtually no fat, so there's no excuse for not including them in your diet. Eat them raw or cooked, in soups, stews and salads, or whizz them up with other fruits and vegetables to make delicious smoothies and juices.

On the outside

Carrot extracts, rich in skin-friendly betacarotene, are added to many cleansers, moisturizing creams, body butters, shampoos and conditioners. You can make your own beauty treatments, too:

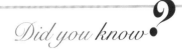

Did you know?

Drinking carrot juice is an ancient remedy to improve healing of wounds, acne, facial redness and scars. Carrot juice is also relatively high in sugar, however, so try to limit yourself to one glass (200 ml/7 fl oz) of this healing nectar per day.

Beauty secrets

● Make a face mask to help your skin glow (also great for oily skin) by mixing grated carrot with honey. Leave on for 15–20 minutes before rinsing. (For dry skin, add a few drops of macadamia, avocado, evening primrose, wheatgerm or argan oil before applying.)
● Help clear blemishes by applying carrot pulp or juice to spots.
● Improve hair shine and treat split ends by adding a few drops of carrot seed essential oil to your shampoo or conditioner, or rubbing directly onto split ends.

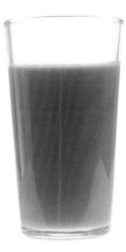

ORANGE ALERT!

Over-consumption of carrots can mimic a cheap fake tan. Although not harmful, it's not a good look, so don't overdo it! This is less likely if you eat raw carrots, rather than over-indulging in carrot juice, when it's easy to consume the equivalent of a whole bunch without realizing!

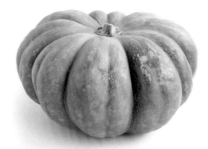

Pumpkins offer many beauty benefits, whether you eat the flesh, seeds or seed oil. They are a rich source of antioxidant pigments and phytoestrogens, which have anti-ageing benefits for skin, helping to maintain collagen levels, especially for older women.

Pumpkins are packed with vitamins (C, E, K) and minerals such as magnesium, zinc and iron. These nutrients help to improve skin tone, promote wound healing, discourage blemishes and boost skin cell renewal.

On the inside

Promote beauty sleep Pumpkin seed extracts are rich in tryptophan – a building block for the hormone melatonin, which helps you sleep. Clinical trials show it significantly improves sleep patterns, with 39 per cent less time awake during the night compared with inactive placebo. Good-quality sleep, and waking feeling refreshed, will improve puffiness and dark circles beneath your eyes.

Combat hair loss and oily skin

Pumpkin seed oil has an ability to inhibit the enzyme 5-alpha reductase, which converts testosterone to the stronger dihydrotestosterone (DHT). This conversion to DHT occurs in hair follicles and is associated with increased oil production, acne and both male- and female-pattern hair loss. Anything that helps to reduce this enzyme is a great beauty tool for reviving oily skin and thinning hair!

In your diet Pumpkin can be enjoyed in both savoury and sweet dishes, as a warming soup or in pasta dishes, in a curry or in a pie, or simply roasted in the oven. Pumpkin seed oil has a lovely nutty flavour and makes a delicious salad dressing or marinade (don't heat it, however, as it has a low smoke point, which makes it unsuitable for frying and means it loses much of its nutritional value).

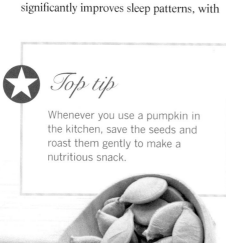

★ *Top tip*

Whenever you use a pumpkin in the kitchen, save the seeds and roast them gently to make a nutritious snack.

On the outside

Pumpkin seed oil is included in many skincare products, including lotions, creams, serums and body washes, as it is softening, moisturizing and a rich source of anti-inflammatory antioxidants and beneficial fatty acids.

The seed oil is also used during professional facials, to soften the skin and make it more receptive to other products. Masks made from pumpkin flesh are rich in antioxidants, help to fade age spots and combat wrinkles, as well as having a gentle exfoliating action to 'dissolve away' dry surface skin cells, reduce pore size and blackheads, and control excess oiliness.

In addition, seed oil is often added to hair products to moisturize and protect hair proteins, hydrate a dry scalp, and to inhibit the formation of DHT within hair follicles.

Beauty secrets

● Add lustre and shine to your hair by applying a drop of pumpkin seed oil to your hair along with your conditioner.
● Make a moisturizing foundation: professional make-up artists mix serums containing pumpkin seed oil with powder mineral foundation to make a customized foundation with moisturizing properties.
● Make a quick rejuvenating mask to tone your skin by mixing 2–3 tablespoons of honey with 1 teaspoon of pumpkin seed oil. Leave on for 10–20 minutes, then rinse.

Pumpkins are packed with vitamins …

PLAN AHEAD

Make a batch of mask mixture and freeze it in an ice-cube tray, so you've got some on tap for future use – just defrost one or two cubes per application, depending on how thickly you like to apply it. To make the mask, simply puree together some ripe, orange pumpkin flesh with a little natural yogurt or honey and a few drops of pumpkin seed oil (if you want an exfoliating effect, add some ground almonds). Apply to the face for 5–10 minutes, then rinse for soft, clean skin.

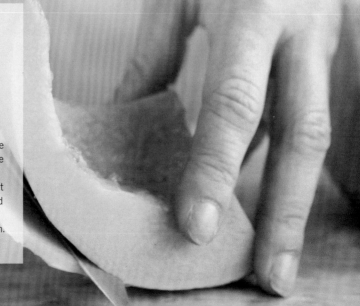

23 *Sweet potatoes*

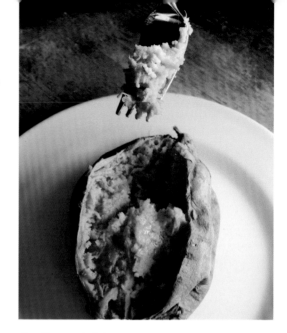

Available in several varieties, those with a moist, orange flesh are the most beneficial, providing a rich source of antioxidant carotenoids and oestrogen-like plant hormones – an anti-ageing wonder food for our skin and hair.

Sweet potatoes also provide useful amounts of magnesium, vitamins C and E, calcium, iron, copper, zinc, manganese, folate and selenium.

On the inside

The oestrogen-like hormones present in sweet potatoes are classed as lignans. These are activated by bowel bacteria to produce numerous beneficial effects on the body, reducing inflammation, boosting healing and having an anti-ageing effect on skin and hair.

Lignans inhibit an enzyme called 5-alpha reductase, which is needed to convert testosterone to the stronger dihydrotestosterone (DHT) linked with hair loss and thinning (see also Pumpkin, page 56). Studies suggest that high intakes are associated with a reduced rate of hair loss – and potentially with hair regeneration. As DHT is also associated with increased oil production and acne, eating sweet potato may also help to protect against these.

In your diet Eat sweet potatoes as you would normal potatoes – baked, mashed or added to vegetable soups, stews and casseroles.

On the outside

Cooked sweet potatoes mash easily and are a popular ingredient in anti-ageing face masks. Sweet-potato masks can also be used as a conditioner for dull, dry hair: simply apply after shampooing, then rinse well, to improve hydration and natural shine.

Beauty secrets

● **Reduce dark circles and puffiness** by placing very thin slices of chilled sweet potato over your eyes. Leave on for 10–20 minutes.
● **Make an antioxidant face toner:** cut half a peeled sweet potato into chunks and boil in a little water for 15–20 minutes until soft. Drain and reserve the liquid to use as a toner (you can use the potato flesh for a mask – see below).
● **For a rejuvenating mask:** mash or blend the cooled sweet potato with 1 tablespoon of honey and 1 tablespoon of Greek yogurt. If you have dry skin, add a teaspoon of your favourite oil, too. Apply to your face and leave for 15 minutes before rinsing.

Red bell peppers

Although bell peppers (also known as capsicum or sweet peppers) come in a variety of colours, the red ones not only taste the sweetest but contain the most vitamins, minerals, antioxidants and polyphenols, too.

Their red colour comes from a mix of over thirty carotenoid pigments, including lycopene, lutein and zeaxanthin, which protect the fruit from sun damage. Red peppers are also one the richest fruit sources of vitamin C, supplying almost three times as much as oranges, weight for weight.

On the inside

As well as being important for collagen production in the skin, vitamin C is a powerful antioxidant that helps to protect skin against sun damage. Women over the age of forty who have higher intakes of vitamin C have been shown to have fewer skin wrinkles and less dryness than those with low intakes, for example.

In your diet Although often eaten cooked, red bell peppers are best eaten raw to obtain the full benefits of the antioxidants they contain, such as vitamin C, which is rapidly destroyed by heat. Add them to salads and sandwich fillings, or cut them into sticks to munch on as a healthy snack.

On the outside

Though it may not be the most obvious choice for a beauty treatment, red peppers can be used to make a very effective mask for your skin.

Beauty secrets

● **For an anti-ageing, antioxidant boost,** place the chopped flesh of one red pepper (discarding the stalk and seeds) in a blender and whizz it up with 1 tablespoon of honey, 1 tablespoon of oatmeal and 5 ml of your favourite oil (such as coconut, avocado, rosehip or wheatgerm oil). Apply to your face for 15 minutes, then rinse.

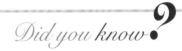

Did you know?

Red peppers have over ten times more betacarotene and 50 per cent more vitamin C than green peppers. So remember: red is best!

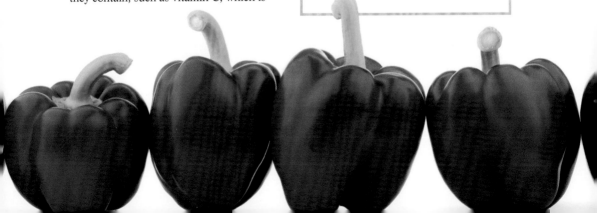

25 Cucumber

Cucumber is 96 per cent water, yet still provides an astonishing array of beauty benefits. Both as part of your diet and as a beauty treatment, this unassuming fruit should be a key component of your beauty regime.

On the inside

Cucumber rind is one of the richest food sources of silica – a mineral that plays an important role in maintaining healthy hair, skin and nails. So don't peel your cucumber before you eat it! Silica is present in such high concentrations in order to protect the cucumber from powdery mildew, which it is susceptible to due to its high water content.

Cucumber juice provides potassium (which flushes excess sodium and fluid to reduce puffiness), magnesium (which fights fatigue), vitamin C (needed for healthy gums and skin) and vitamin K (involved in blood clotting and which, when applied to the skin, can reduce thread veins and bruising).

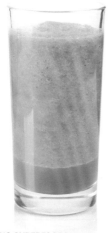

Cucumber mint smoothie

Place half a chopped cucumber in a blender together with 250 ml (½ pt) coconut water, 1 sprig mint leaves, 1 ripe kiwi (peeled) and a few spinach leaves (you won't taste them but they provide additional nutrients and colour). Whizz until smooth. Add crushed ice and sweeten with stevia – a natural calorie-free sweetener – if desired.

In your diet Add cucumber to your salads, sandwiches and wraps, and experiment with cucumber soup and cucumber smoothies. You can even add it to stir-fries and curries.

On the outside

Cucumbers were first cultivated in India over ten thousand years ago, and the Romans, too, were well aware of their benefits, inventing an early form of greenhouse to ensure a year-round supply. Beauticians in ancient times would use them to make a brightening skin tonic to fade freckles, tighten fine lines and reduce cellulite.

Here are just some of the ways you can incorporate cucumber in your own beauty routine:

Soothe puffy eyes Cut two slices from a chilled cucumber. Lie down, place one

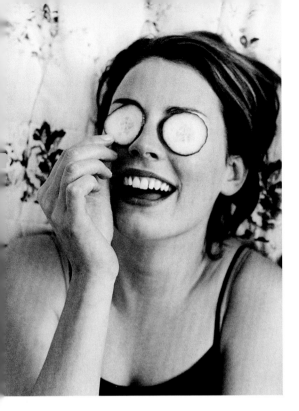

Caution

Though rare, some people are allergic to cucumber proteins. Patch-test a small area of skin by applying a cucumber ring for 15 minutes to ensure there is no reddening or itching.

slice of cucumber over each closed eye and relax for 15 minutes. This constricts blood vessels, to reduce underlying puffiness while hydrating parched skin. Regular use helps to reduce eye bags and dark circles.

Tone your skin Blend half a chopped cucumber, 45 ml (1½ fl oz) witch hazel and 30 ml (1 fl oz) filtered/mineral water until smooth. Pass the mixture through a fine-mesh sieve or squeeze through cheesecloth to remove the solids (save the solids and use them for a 5-minute face mask). Pour the liquid into a clean screw-top bottle and apply with a cotton-wool pad as required. This brightens, refreshes and tones skin, as well as tightening enlarged pores.

Zap a blemish Mix a small amount of cucumber juice (grate some cucumber and squeeze to obtain the juice) with an equal amount of lemon juice. Apply to spots for 15 minutes, then wash off. (If you have dry rather than oily skin, add a little manuka honey, too.) This will shrink spots and reduce inflammation and redness.

After-sun treatment If your skin is parched and sore from too much sun, cucumber juice can cool and soothe the affected area. (Sunscreen and sensible sun-exposure times will prevent burning, so this remedy should only be used as a last resort!)

For a refreshing bath Add a handful of Dead Sea salts, one sliced cucumber and a few drops of diluted essential oils (see note below) to a warm bath, and lie back and relax for 15–20 minutes, preferably in candlelight.
NOTE: Most essential oils should be diluted before coming in contact with your skin. Add 5 drops to a tablespoon of carrier oil (such as almond or avocado) and mix. Choose a single favourite oil, or a blend of up to three (for example, 1 drop rose, 2 drops lemon, 2 drops vanilla).

26 *Tomatoes*

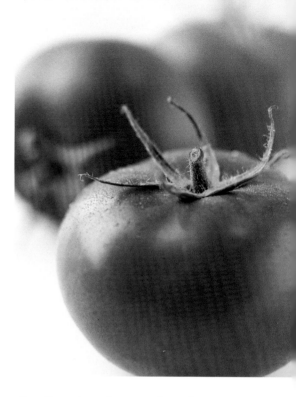

Tomatoes help to protect our skin against sun damage, as well as reducing oxidation of 'bad' LDL-cholesterol, helping to maintain a healthy blood-delivery boost to your hair, skin and nails.

The vibrant red colour of tomatoes comes from an antioxidant pigment called lycopene, which protects the fruit from sun damage. Tomato lycopene can offer the same protection to your skin, reducing the adverse ageing effects of ultraviolet light.

On the inside

Lycopene is normally locked away inside tomato cells, so you absorb far less from raw tomatoes than cooked. Cooked tomatoes release *five times* more of this vital nutrient, which means some of the richest dietary sources include tomato ketchup, concentrated tomato puree/paste and passata (pizza sauce). And if you drizzle your tomato soup or pizza with olive oil, you boost lycopene absorption threefold, as it is highly fat-soluble.

A substance extracted from the jelly of tomatoes, known as 'Fruitflow', has been found to protect against abnormal blood clotting and contribute to a healthy blood flow, vital for healthy skin and hair. Tomatoes are also rich in vitamin C, which boosts collagen production to help protect against wrinkles.

Protect your skin Researchers from Newcastle University in the UK compared the skin of women eating 5 tablespoons (55 g/2 oz) tomato paste plus 10 g (¹/₃ oz) olive oil every day, for twelve weeks, with a similar group taking just the olive oil as a supplement. They were exposed to UV rays at the beginning and end of the

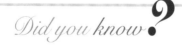

Did you know?

Most people obtain less than 1 mg lycopene per day, yet you need at least six times this amount for health circulatory benefits. Aim to consume 200 ml (7 fl oz) tomato juice, 150 g (5 oz) tomato sauce or one lycopene tablet a day – and don't feel guilty when adding tomato ketchup to your plate!

trial, and it was found those eating tomato paste developed 33 per cent less redness, suggesting this simple dietary step offered a sun protection factor (SPF) equivalent to 1.3. Skin biopsies also showed increased skin levels of procollagen, which improves elasticity, in those consuming tomato paste, and less damage to skin mitochondrial DNA, which is linked to skin ageing.

On the outside

Tomatoes are a rich source of complexion-brightening fruit acids that help to combat oiliness, tighten pores, exfoliate dead cells, reduce blackheads and discourage blemishes …

Beauty secrets

● Rub a tomato wedge over your face for 5 minutes, just before you go to bed, then rinse.
● For an all-over facial, slice a tomato thinly, lie back and arrange the sliced tomatoes over your face. Relax for 10 minutes, then rinse and pat dry.
● Help heal blemishes by applying a dab of tomato paste from a tube to spots.
● Make a cool, soothing mask to soften your skin by mixing 1 tablespoon of tomato paste with 1 tablespoon of natural yogurt. Leave on for 15 minutes, then rinse.
● Shrink pores by mixing 1 tablespoon of fresh tomato juice with 1 teaspoon of fresh lemon or lime juice and massage into affected areas using a cotton-wool pad. Leave on for 15 minutes, then rinse.
● Treat dandruff by applying tomato pulp to your scalp for 30 minutes before shampooing.

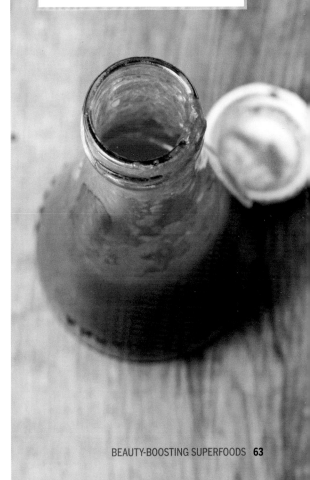

Easy tomato sauce

Fill a baking tray with halved tomatoes, add some garlic and fresh or dried herbs, drizzle with olive oil and roast in the oven (on a low to medium heat) for 30 minutes. Once cooked, liquidize and use as a base for soups, stews and pasta sauces. (It's a good idea to make large batches – especially when tomatoes are plentiful and cheap – and freeze in separate portions for future use.)

Green leafy vegetables

Green leafy vegetables, such as spring greens, spinach, watercress, parsley and curly kale, are a rich source of folate, a B vitamin needed for protein and DNA synthesis in rapidly dividing cells, such as those found in the skin.

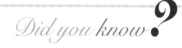
Green leaves are also a good vegetarian source of iron, which transports oxygen around the body for healthy hair, skin and nails, and vitamin C, which boosts iron absorption. Spinach and curly kale in particular are an excellent source of calcium, needed for strong bones and teeth, and carotenoid antioxidants, which protect your skin from the inflammatory effects of ultraviolet light.

Green leafy vegetables also contain substances called indoles that promote the metabolism of oestrogen. They help to protect against skin ageing when oestrogen levels start to fall as the menopause approaches.

On the inside

Folate helps lower levels of homocysteine, an amino acid which has been linked with skin depigmentation in vitiligo. Treatment with folic acid (the synthetic form of folate) plus vitamin B_{12}, together with safe, sensible exposure to the sun, can help skin to redevelop pigmentation. In one study involving 100 people, repigmentation occurred in 52 per cent, and was most evident on sun-exposed areas.

Improve complexion and reduce wrinkles In a study carried out on female volunteers aged between twenty-three and fifty-eight, each volunteer was asked to include one bag of raw watercress (80 g/3 oz) in their normal daily diet for four weeks. Their complexions were then extensively analysed for wrinkles, texture, UV spots, redness and levels of bacteria. Ten out of eleven experienced visible improvements and, in one case, facial wrinkles improved by as much as 39 per cent. The watercress was eaten raw in salads, sandwiches and smoothies, or just wilted into pasta.

Combat ageing Research involving 400 people aged over seventy found that those with a high intake of green leafy vegetables showed 21 per cent fewer signs of skin ageing and wrinkling than those with low intakes.

EAT YOUR GREENS!

The body stores very little folate, and dietary lack rapidly causes deficiency; it is one of the most widespread vitamin deficiencies in developed countries. So make sure greens are a staple component of your diet!

In your diet Prolonged boiling destroys much of the folate and vitamin C present in green leafy vegetables, so try to eat leaves raw or only lightly steamed, to preserve their nutrients.

On the outside

An antioxidant plant hormone called kinetin, derived from green leaves, promotes growth and has an anti-ageing effect on plants. It is now included in many anti-ageing creams, after studies showed it helps to reduce areas of hyperpigmentation (age spots), improve skin texture, colour, blotchiness and fine wrinkles, as well as stimulating the proliferation of new, healthy skin cells. Kinetin, applied twice a day, strengthens the skin barrier to reduce water evaporation from skin by 26 per cent. This improvement in hydration helps skin feel plumper and more youthful.

Kinetin creams are also helpful for people with rosacea, which causes redness and acne-like facial blemishes. Topical kinetin at a strength of just 0.1 per cent has been found to reduce redness, skin texture and mottling.

Beauty secrets

● Make a refreshing and rejuvenating face mask by blending a bag of spinach with a little water to make a paste. Apply to the face, leave for 20 minutes, then rinse.

Spinach smoothie

Blend together 250 ml (1/2 pt) apple juice, a bag of spinach and the flesh from half an avocado, and drink while fresh!

28 *Reishi mushrooms*

Revered in China, Japan, Korea and Tibet for over 2,500 years, reishi mushrooms are traditionally used to boost physical and mental energy levels, to promote vitality and longevity, and to boost immunity.

The Japanese term 'reishi' means 'spiritual mushroom', while in China it is known as 'ling zhi' – the mushroom of immortality. Of the six different colours of reishi mushroom (green, black, white, red, yellow and rare purple), Red Reishi (*Ganoderma lucidum*) is considered the most potent.

Too woody, fibrous and bitter to eat, it is widely consumed in the form of teas and herbal supplements. Reishi contains at least a hundred different triterpenes, which are structurally similar to steroid hormones, including a unique group of ganoderic acids that possess regenerative properties.

Reishi mycelium consists of the white mushroom 'roots' that grow into wood to extract nutrients. Periodically, the mycelium develops the fruiting mushroom on its surface. While reishi mycelium was not traditionally used as a tonic herb, scientists have discovered it is a richer source of the same active polysaccharides as the mushroom itself, making it significantly cheaper to produce in the form of tablets and capsules.

On the inside

Reishi is one of the most widely researched Asian medicinal plants, with a variety of beneficial uses.

Combat eye bags and dark circles

Reishi increases blood flow to the brain to enhance energy levels and gives a more restful night's sleep. Those who take reishi regularly enjoy a deep, refreshing

---

Caution

While there appears to be no cross-sensitivity with traditional 'button' mushrooms, and reishi can usually be taken by those allergic to field mushrooms, check with your doctor first if you do have a pre-existing mushroom allergy.

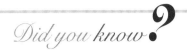
sleep, and a Zen-like sense of calm. It is especially helpful during times of stress and fatigue, when reishi can produce significant improvements in sleep and overall well-being within eight weeks.

Slow premature ageing Laboratory studies have found that extracts improve cell regeneration and increase cellular resistance to the ageing effects of toxins. In the East, reishi is used to slow premature ageing and research suggests that, as well as acting as an antioxidant, mushroom extracts can block the effects of enzymes such as elastase, which break down collagen during the ageing process.

Reduce skin inflammation Reishi is also used to treat skin rashes such as eczema and rosacea, due to its anti-inflammatory properties, and to reduce acne through immune and antibacterial actions.

Condition hair By boosting blood flow to the peripheries, Reishi promotes the growth of healthy, glossy hair, plumps skin and strengthens nails. It is an ancient Chinese remedy to reduce premature hair loss and baldness, and is said to help prevent premature hair-greying.

Recommended dose 500 mg mycelium extracts, two to three times daily.

On the outside

Reishi is included in several high-end, anti-ageing creams – and often used in spa treatments – for its skin-rejuvenating properties. These include facial serums, night creams and eye creams, as well as beauty masks.

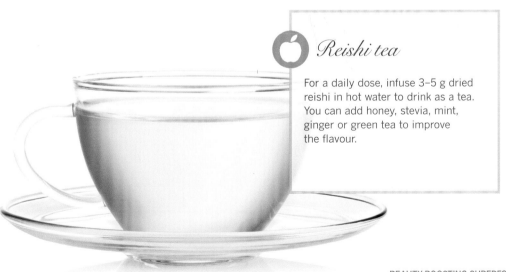

Reishi tea

For a daily dose, infuse 3–5 g dried reishi in hot water to drink as a tea. You can add honey, stevia, mint, ginger or green tea to improve the flavour.

29 *Beansprouts*

Sprouting legumes are one of the most nutritious foods, packed full of amino acids, vitamins, minerals and essential fatty acids – and great for your nails, skin and hair!

Beansprouts are a rich source of plant hormones which have an oestrogen-like action in the body. These interact with receptors in your hair, skin and nails to stimulate collagen production and help to maintain skin texture, tone and hydration in later life. Beansprouts are also a good source of vitamins B_1, B_2, B_3 and folate, which is vital for rapidly dividing cells

such as those producing new hair, skin and nails. They also provide vitamin C, which acts as an antioxidant and boosts collagen production, plus iron, zinc and selenium for healthy hair and scalp.

Because they are actively growing, beansprouts provide up to one hundred times as many active enzymes as are normally found in fruit and vegetables.

On the inside

Research comparing dietary intakes with degrees of skin wrinkling in elderly people living in Greece, Australia and Sweden found that those with good intakes of legumes, such as beansprouts, showed 11 per cent fewer signs of skin ageing than

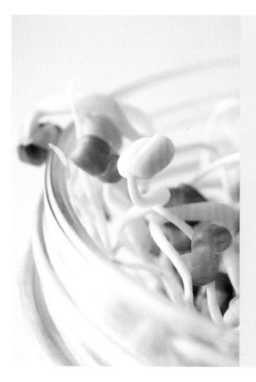

GROW YOUR OWN

Beansprouts are easy to grow at home, in jam jars or customized germinators which provide the correct conditions of warmth and humidity for optimal growth. Simply rinse 4–6 tablespoons of mixed organic seeds in water, then sprinkle lightly over a germinator or add to a glass jar, and allow to germinate for three to five days.

Always use certified organic seed that is GM-free and non-irradiated, from reputable food-crop suppliers (make sure the seeds are labelled as suitable for sprouting). This minimizes the risk of food poisoning due to *E.coli* or salmonella contamination during seed production. Children, seniors and those with weak immune systems may choose not to consume raw sprouts.

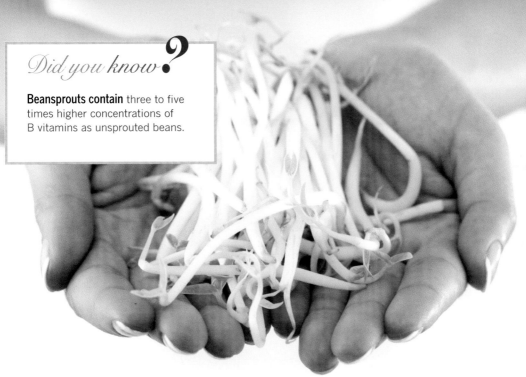

Beansprouts are best eaten raw for maximum benefit.

those with low intakes. Eating beansprouts daily is also said to help reduce hair thinning and hair loss.

In your diet Beansprouts are best eaten raw, to preserve their enzymes. Add to salads or smoothies, or, if including them in stir-fries, add them at the last minute, so they merely warm through (the enzymes break down and become inactive at temperatures above 43°C/110°F). Home-sprouted seeds add a delicious, nutrient-rich crunch to your diet. Suitable seeds

to sprout include alfalfa, soy, radish, mung bean, broccoli, fenugreek, gram, white radish, red clover, wheat, lentil, quinoa, mustard, cress (see box opposite). The highest oestrogenic activity is found in sprouting red clover, mung beans, alfalfa and soy beans.

On the outside

Mung-bean beauty masks are widely used in Asia as an anti-ageing, anti-freckle and anti-blemish treatment. The enzymes present help to reduce dark spots and brighten skin tone.

Beauty secrets
● **Make a home-made mask** by blending together a few tablespoons of sprouted beans with a similar volume of natural bio yogurt. Apply to skin and rinse after 15 minutes.

30 Edamame beans

These green, immature soy beans, picked before they ripen, are rich in oestrogen-like plant hormones called isoflavones, which do wonders for our skin and help protect against wrinkles.

Edamame – the Japanese term for 'stem beans' – are eaten raw, boiled or steamed. The isoflavones they contain have a similar structure to human oestradiol and, although their effect is a hundredfold weaker, they provide a significant oestrogen boost for women whose own levels are falling due to the menopause. Edamame beans are also a good source of vitamins (B, C, K and folate), as well as the minerals manganese, magnesium, iron and zinc.

On the inside

Human oestrogen is made up of three different hormones – oestriol, oestrone and oestradiol – which have effects throughout the body. In the skin, they boost production of collagen protein and promote skin thickness, elasticity and hydration. As oestrogen levels fall in the years leading up to the menopause, skin tends to become thinner, with dryness, itching, slackness and wrinkling. These effects are hastened by the damaging effects of sunlight.

Top tip

To increase your intake of other types of oestrogen-like plant hormones, aim to eat more chickpeas, lentils, exotic members of the cruciferous family such as Chinese leaves and kohlrabi, plus nuts, seeds and wholegrains.

Isoflavones present in edamame beans and other soy products provide an oestrogen hormone boost to help keep your skin firm and smooth. By boosting collagen production, damping down inflammation and guarding against the UV damage that causes collagen to degrade, a diet that is plentiful in isoflavones helps to protect against wrinkles.

Isoflavones present in soy beans are mostly in an inactive form, bound to a glycoside sugar. When you eat them, they are broken down by intestinal bacteria to release the active plant hormones genistein, daidzein and glycitein. Some people naturally possess sufficient probiotic intestinal bacteria to metabolize daidzein to a more powerful oestrogen called equol, which is also a potent antioxidant. However, as there is no way of knowing whether you fall into this category, it's a good idea to eat live bio yogurt and to take a probiotic supplement, to ensure you gain the maximum benefit from eating edamame soy beans.

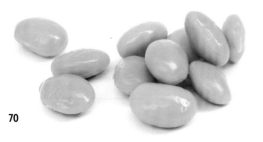

Isoflavones present in edamame beans help keep your skin firm and smooth.

Boost radiance and combat wrinkles In Japan, where soy is a dietary staple, intakes of isoflavones are 50–100 mg per day for both men and women, compared with typical Western intakes of just 2–5 mg per day. Blood levels of isoflavones in Japan are therefore as much as 110 times higher than those typically found in the West, which may explain why Japanese women are renowned for their beautiful skin and lack of significant wrinkles. Preliminary studies suggest that dietary isoflavones help to protect skin against sun damage and improve radiance, while reducing wrinkle formation and hair loss.

Recommended dose Isoflavone supplements are usually taken at a dose of 40–100 mg per day.

In your diet Edamame are now widely available frozen and can be added to soups, stews, bean salads, risottos, or mashed with avocado and a little healthy nut oil to make a healthy dip. They are also often served in the pod as a healthy snack at Japanese restaurants, though avoid those served with salt – ask for a spicy sauce or eat them plain instead.

On the outside

In China, home-made soy bean masks have been used for thousands of years to cleanse the skin, improve firmness, reverse sun damage and prevent premature wrinkles. Try making your own to use at home …

Beauty secrets
● Rejuvenate your skin: blend a handful of edamame with 1 teaspoon of sweet almond or jojoba oil to make a paste. Add an egg white and 1 teaspoonful of honey. Leave for 5 minutes to set, then add 1 tablespoon of oatmeal. Apply to your skin, leave on for 20 minutes, then rinse off, rubbing gently to exfoliate dead skin cells.

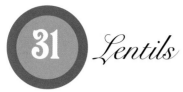

31 *Lentils*

Lentils provide protein, fibre, B vitamins and minerals such as magnesium, iron, copper, zinc and selenium, important for healthy skin, hair and nails and for combating the signs of ageing.

This edible legume is available in a variety of colours, from red, green and brown to yellow or black varieties (red and orange lentils also provide a small amount of antioxidant carotenoid pigment). They are also a rich source of two types of oestrogen-like plant hormones – mainly lignans, plus useful amounts of isoflavones.

On the inside

Falling oestrogen levels, as the menopause approaches, cause skin to thin and become increasingly dry, itchy, sallow and slack, which contributes to the development of wrinkles. Lentils interact with human oestrogen receptors to provide a useful oestrogen boost, to postpone these effects.

Studies have also found that those with a good dietary intake of legumes like lentils show 11 per cent fewer signs of skin ageing than those consuming only small amounts.

In your diet Include lentils in soups, stews or casseroles, or bake a lentil loaf – the perfect hormone boost for older women in the run-up to the menopause.

On the outside

In India, lentil face masks are commonly used to help keep skin soft and supple, and to discourage wrinkles.

Beauty secrets

● **For an anti-ageing mask,** soak some red lentils in water overnight, then blend the drained lentils with a little rosehip or coconut oil to make a smooth paste. Apply to clean, dry skin and leave for 15 minutes before rinsing.

● **To reduce skin oiliness,** soak some black lentils in water overnight, then blend the drained lentils with 1 teaspoon of fuller's earth, plus half a teaspoon of freshly squeezed lime juice, to make a thick paste. Apply to clean, dry skin and leave for 15 minutes before rinsing.

Did you know?

Lentils are used to make dhal, which, when served with rice, helps provide a balanced intake of the amino acids needed for healthy hair follicles.

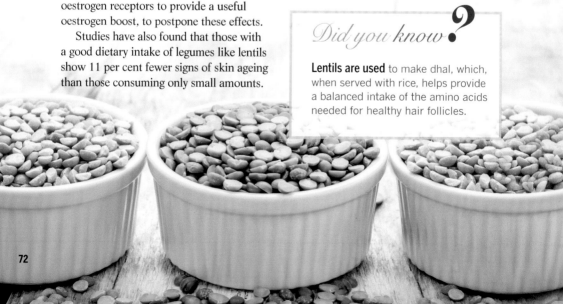

32 *Honey*

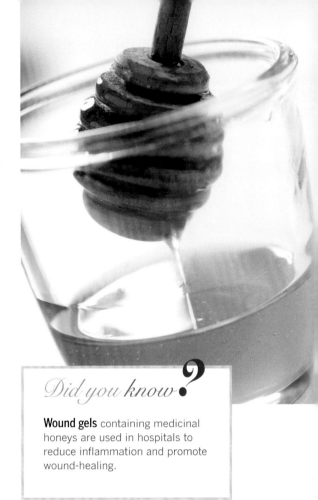

Honey is one of the oldest known beauty treatments, used by the Ancient Egyptians to soften skin and lighten uneven pigmentation. They also used it during embalming, thanks to its preservative qualities.

All honeys absorb fluid due to their high concentration of natural sugars. This osmotic effect makes it difficult for bacteria to thrive. Most also release natural antiseptics, such as hydrogen peroxide and gluconic acid. Honey made from medicinal flowers such as the manuka, or New Zealand tea tree, has unique antibacterial properties against over 250 types of bacteria – including antibiotic-resistant strains such as MRSA (methicillin-resistant Staphylococcus aureus).

On the outside

Pamper your skin and hair with these home remedies:

Beauty secrets

● **To give oily skin a treat,** clean and dry your face, then spread a dollop of raw honey over it. Rinse after 15 minutes.
● **For dry skin,** add 1 tablespoon of your

Did you know?

Wound gels containing medicinal honeys are used in hospitals to reduce inflammation and promote wound-healing.

favourite oil – evening primrose, rosehip or coconut – to a dollop of honey and blend. Use as above.
● **To add softness and shine to dull, dry hair,** add 1 teaspoon of honey to your shampoo. Wash and lather as normal. For a more intensive treatment, apply a post-shampoo conditioner made by mixing 1 tablespoon of raw honey with 2 tablespoons of coconut or argan oil. Apply to the ends of your hair, cover with a shower cap or hot towel for 15 minutes, then rinse well.

Caution

Although honey is an excellent treatment for blemishes, it's important not to put 'normal' honey on wounds. Use a sterile, medicinal honey gel from a pharmacy.

33 *Green tea*

Green tea is packed with highly powerful antioxidants that have a general anti-ageing effect on the circulation and skin. It boosts the rate at which the body burns calories, too.

Green tea is produced from the young leaves and leaf buds of *Camellia sinensis* – the same shrub that produces black tea. While black tea is made by crushing and fermenting freshly cut tea leaves so they oxidize before drying, green tea is made by steaming and drying the fresh tea leaves immediately after harvesting. Over 30 per cent of the dry weight of green tea leaves consists of powerful flavonoid antioxidants such as catechins, and these antioxidants are at least a hundred times more powerful than vitamin C, and twenty-five times more powerful than vitamin E.

Green tea is also an excellent healthy source of caffeine, which is increasingly used in cosmetics, as it is readily absorbed through the skin.

On the inside

The caffeine found in green tea acts as a mild stimulant to improve concentration. It also dilates blood vessels to improve blood flow to hair follicles, skin and nails.

Improve skin elasticity In a trial involving forty women, those taking green tea extracts and using a green tea cream showed significant improvement in skin elasticity within eight weeks.

Combat wrinkles In a wide-ranging study comparing dietary intakes with degree of skin wrinkling, those with a high tea consumption showed an astonishing 54 per cent fewer signs of skin wrinkling than those with a low intake.

Lose weight Green tea extracts boost the rate at which you burn calories by as much as 40 per cent over a 24-hour period, by increasing heat release (thermogenesis) as well as blocking the activity of intestinal enzymes needed to absorb dietary fat. Several trials suggest that adding green tea extracts to a weight loss regime helps to improve fat loss; for example, a study involving sixty obese adults following a prepared diet of three meals a day found that those taking green tea extracts lost an additional 2.7 kg (6 lb) during the first month, 5.1 kg (11 lb) during the second month and 3.3 kg (7 lb) during the third month.

Recommended dose Drink four cups of green tea daily, or take supplements of 500 mg daily (standardized to contain at least 50 per cent polyphenols).

On the outside

Green tea antioxidants are included in many commercially produced cosmetic products as they offer several different benefits:

Soothe sunburn When applied topically, green tea antioxidants help to protect cells from UV radiation, decreasing UV-

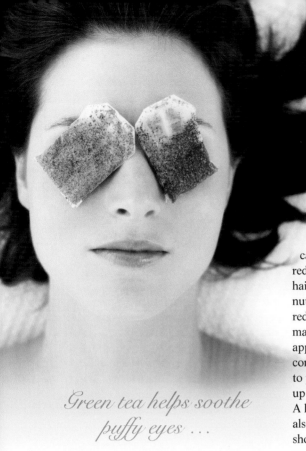

Green tea helps soothe puffy eyes ...

extracts increase blood flow through tiny capillaries, stimulate the breakdown of fat deposits and prevent excessive accumulation of fat within cells. By stimulating lymph drainage, it also improves the removal of released fatty acids and toxins.

Stimulate hair growth Green tea caffeine stimulates scalp hair growth by reducing smooth muscle tension around hair follicles to improve blood flow and nutrient delivery. It also inhibits 5-alpha reductase, an enzyme associated with both male- and female-pattern hair loss. When applied as a shampoo, just 2 minutes' contact with the scalp allows the caffeine to penetrate deeply, where it remains for up to 48 hours, even after hair-washing. A leave-on caffeine combination that also includes vitamins B_3 and B_5 has been shown to increase the cross-sectional area of scalp hair fibres by 10 per cent, to produce noticeable thickening. Caffeinated shampoos are especially helpful for women over the age of forty and men with thinning hair.

induced redness and DNA damage to slow photo-ageing of the skin. Preliminary evidence suggests extracts can improve hyperpigmentation and fine lines.

Alleviate rosacea Green tea extracts help to reduce inflammation and protect against sun-induced flare-ups.

Ease eye puffiness Caffeine stimulates blood flow and, when applied as a gel to delicate tissues around the eyes, can help to reduce puffiness.

Combat cellulite When included in anti-cellulite products, green tea caffeine

Beauty secrets
- **Soothe puffy eyes** by placing cooled, used green tea bags over your eyes (save the bags when you make a cup of tea and store them in the fridge).
- **Make an exfoliating scrub** by mixing cooled green tea with oatmeal.
- **Boost hair shine and stimulate hair growth** by using cooled green tea (soaked overnight) as a hair rinse. Leave on for 10 minutes, massaging your scalp, then rinse.

34 Dark chocolate

Cocoa solids contain more antioxidants than just about any other food – there are over 25,000 antioxidant units in a single spoonful of raw cocoa powder! – helping to combat the signs of premature ageing.

Just 40 g (1½ oz) of dark chocolate provides more than 300 mg of super-protective polyphenols known as oligomer flavonoids. These have beneficial effects on the circulation, helping to dilate blood vessels and boost the supply of oxygen and nutrients to hair follicles, skin and nails. They also have anti-ageing effects that may protect against premature wrinkles. In addition, cocoa powder is a good source of minerals, including calcium, copper, magnesium and zinc, which are needed for healthy hair, skin and nails.

On the inside

Research from the *Journal of Cosmetic Dermatology* shows that regular consumption of dark chocolate helps to protect the skin from the harmful effects of ultraviolet radiation, to reduce premature skin ageing. Another study, in the *Journal of Nutrition*, found that dark chocolate also improves skin thickness and hydration, both of which are important for healthier, younger-looking skin.

Combat acne and eczema Although it is often claimed that chocolate makes acne worse, there is no consistent evidence that this is the case. In fact, dark chocolate

containing at least 72 per cent cocoa solids might be expected to *improve* inflammatory skin problems, due to the antioxidants present. Scientists have recently found that probiotic gut bacteria can break down indigestible chocolate compounds into polymers that have an additional, anti-inflammatory action which could help to reduce acne and eczema. The most beneficial effect came from eating 2 tablespoons of cocoa powder per day.

On the outside

The huge number of antioxidants contained cocoa solids help to neutralize the free radicals associated with premature ageing. Dark chocolate is added to many cosmetic products to draw out toxins and promote a

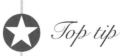

Top tip

If you don't have any ground oatmeal to use in a mask, use rolled oats instead, and pulse the ingredients in a blender.

Dark chocolate improves skin thickness and hydration, important for healthier, younger-looking skin.

smooth, toned complexion. It is also found in shower gels, and body and lip butters. As well as offering beauty benefits, its colour, aroma and creamy texture provide a luxuriant and irresistible touch of glamour.

Beauty secrets

● **Make an anti-ageing face pack** to treat dull, tired skin: blend together 50 ml (1³/₄ oz) natural, unsweetened Greek bio yogurt with 1 tablespoon each of cocoa powder and honey. Apply the mask to your face, leave for 20 minutes, then rinse.

● **Improve the texture and tone of your skin**, whether it's oily, acne-prone, dry, ageing or sensitive, with this home-made chocolate-oat beauty mask: simply blend together 5 tablespoons of cocoa powder, 4 of honey, 3 of ground oatmeal and 2 of Greek bio yogurt, until well combined. Apply to your face, leave for 15–20 minutes, then rinse using a gentle massaging action to exfoliate dead skin cells.

CHOOSING CHOCOLATE

Sadly, not all chocolate is good for you ... White and milk chocolate have a high fat and sugar content, so are best reserved as an occasional treat. Go for dark chocolate containing at least 70 per cent cocoa solids, and use pure cocoa powder.

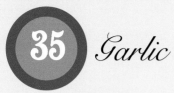

35 Garlic

This popular kitchen herb, with its pungent odour, is perhaps not an obvious beautifier, but the secret lies in its ability to boost the circulation, especially through small arteries (arterioles) and small veins (venules), increasing the blood flow to the skin to impart a healthy glow.

Increased blood flow to scalp follicles helps to promote hair thickness and strength, while improved circulation within the nail beds encourages the growth of strong, less brittle nails. Garlic also has antioxidant, antiseptic, antibacterial and antiviral properties, and a regular intake may help to reduce inflammatory skin conditions such as rosacea, acne, eczema and psoriasis.

On the inside

Cutting or crushing a garlic clove releases a strong-smelling, sulphurous substance called allicin, which has several beneficial effects on the circulation.

Improve nail health By reducing blood stickiness and dilating blood vessels, it improves blood flow to the peripheries, especially to the nails. Garlic extracts have been shown to dilate arterioles and venules to improve blood flow to the skin by almost 50 per cent and to the nail folds by as much as 55 per cent. The effects on blood-vessel dilation can be seen within 5 hours of taking a single dose, and wear off over 24 hours.

Boost skin elasticity and combat sagging As well as boosting blood flow, the sulphur present in garlic (and other

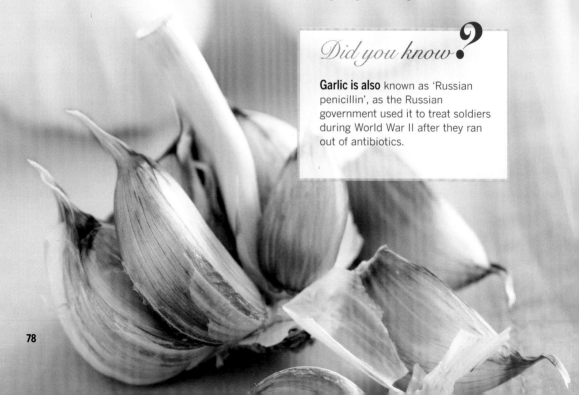

Did you know?

Garlic is also known as 'Russian penicillin', as the Russian government used it to treat soldiers during World War II after they ran out of antibiotics.

members of the onion family) helps to promote the formation of collagen and keratin to strengthen hair, skin and nails. Lack of sulphur is associated with loss of skin elasticity and premature sagging and wrinkling. Researchers have found that those with a high dietary intake of garlic show 20 per cent fewer signs of skin ageing than those with low intakes.

Avoid a red, raw nose! Laboratory research has found that garlic and black garlic extracts increase the activity of immune cells that target both bacterial and viral infections. People taking garlic extracts have significantly fewer colds and, if they do succumb, the duration of symptoms is significantly shorter (in tests, one and a half days, as compared to five days).

In your diet Garlic is best consumed raw, to obtain the maximum benefit from the allicin – however, this is not to everyone's taste! Let your garlic sit for 5–10 minutes after crushing, to allow the allicin to form; this also makes it more stable and resistant to the heat of cooking, though only cook for a short period – no more than 15 minutes – on a low to medium heat, or add towards the end of cooking, if possible, to obtain the most beneficial effects.

Recommended dose For a guaranteed dose of allicin, opt for standardized garlic-powder tablets (ensuring you get the same benefit per dose) – one 600–900 mg tablet daily. Enteric tablet coating reduces garlic odour on the breath and protects the active ingredients from degradation in the stomach.

BLACK GARLIC

Black garlic delivers the same health and beauty benefits as normal garlic, only with significantly less odour. It's produced by a natural fermentation process under carefully controlled conditions of high temperature and humidity, which converts unstable 'smelly' sulphur-containing compounds into stable, odourless substances and also produces a dark pigment, melanoidin, which accounts for its colour. Highly prized by gourmands, it has a soft, savoury-sweet flavour with balsamic and molasses-like undertones.

On the outside

Daily application of the juice from a freshly cut garlic clove is a traditional treatment for warts. An antiviral action kills the wart virus but, if too much garlic is used, the skin will blister, so care is needed. Protect surrounding skin with petroleum jelly, and apply a small test amount initially, in case of an allergic reaction (if it starts to burn, wash off thoroughly straight away).

Some sources suggest squeezing sliced garlic cloves on your scalp and massaging in to boost hair growth, and applying cut garlic to clear a pimple or treat psoriasis and other skin rashes. However, these actions could cause irritation, and will certainly not enhance your personal aroma(!), so you may be advised to stick to consuming garlic fresh or as a supplement to make the most of its benefits.

36 *Chilli peppers*

Not the most obvious of beauty-boosting foods, chilli peppers (also known as cayenne) do offer unique benefits, thanks to a substance they contain called capsaicin.

Caution

Although you can make your own lip-plumper using lip gloss and chopped chillies, this is not recommended, as it's easy to get the quantities wrong and cause extreme discomfort. If you wish to try this effect, go for a commercial lip-plumping product!

The heat in this popular 'hot' culinary spice comes from the capsaicin, which is concentrated in the white tissue supporting the chilli seeds. The hotter the pepper, the higher its capsaicin content. Capsaicin is an irritant that produces a burning sensation when in contact with delicate tissues such as the mucous membranes lining the lip and mouth – but it does have some beneficial effects, too!

On the inside

Capsaicin is a potent antioxidant and has a powerful anti-ageing action in the skin.

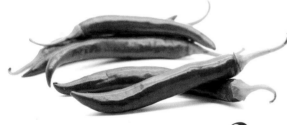

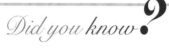

Did you know

The hottest chilli peppers are habanero, followed by Scotch bonnet, the Jamaican hot pepper and Thai peppers (also known as bird's eye). The mildest are sweet bell peppers, which have no detectable heat.

It is able to block the activation of damaging nuclear transcription factors (molecules that control the activity of a gene) that are triggered by exposure to ultraviolet light.

Maintain a healthy weight Studies suggest that capsaicin may have a role in reducing obesity. Capsaicin helps to suppress appetite by increasing sensations of fullness and decreasing the desire to eat. People who regularly eat spicy food containing chillies tend to eat less food overall, and are less likely to become significantly overweight. Capsaicin also blocks fat storage and increases the rate at which fat that has already been stored is burned to produce energy.

On the outside

Chilli pepper extracts are used in some lip-plumping products to give a fuller look. The diluted capsaicin stimulates blood flow to the lips to produce swelling. This usually causes burning sensations and tingling at first, as the capsaicin stimulates special nerve endings that detect pain. The lips then become numb, and a characteristic flare develops as blood vessels dilate. Local blood flow increases and the lips plump up and may feel warm.

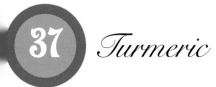

37 *Turmeric*

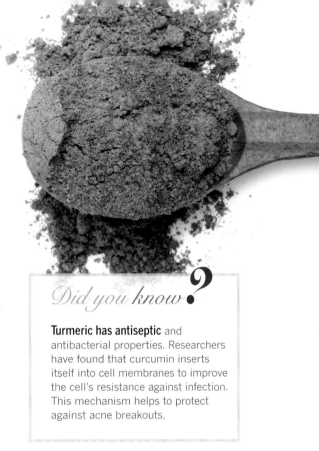

This member of the ginger family, commonly used in Indian cuisine, has a long history of use in Ayurvedic and Chinese medicine for its antioxidant and anti-inflammatory actions. The active ingredient is a yellow pigment known as curcumin.

On the inside

Turmeric boosts liver function and bile production to improve digestion and relieve abdominal bloating.

Recommended dose If taking as a supplement, take 1 g daily.

In your diet Add it to curries or rice dishes, or use it to make tea – add half a teaspoon to 1–2 cups of boiling water, simmer for 10 minutes, strain and add honey or lemon to taste.

On the outside

Antioxidants that neutralize free radicals are important ingredients in anti-ageing skin products. These help to reduce damage from ultraviolet light and other environmental agents, as well as the metabolic processes that set up inflammatory reactions. Inflammation in the skin causes microscars which can progress to blemishes or wrinkles. Curcumin derived from turmeric roots has been shown to increase the activity of genes involved in damping down inflammation, and to help block the activity of destructive enzymes that

Did you know?

Turmeric has antiseptic and antibacterial properties. Researchers have found that curcumin inserts itself into cell membranes to improve the cell's resistance against infection. This mechanism helps to protect against acne breakouts.

break down supporting tissues and hasten skin sagging.

Although curcumin itself is bright yellow, the tetrahydrocurcuminoids derived from it are colourless and are included in cosmetic creams to brighten and lighten.

Beauty secrets

Make a topical treatment to help clear blemishes and reduce oil secretion:
● **For oily skin:** mix some turmeric powder with orange juice to make a paste. Apply to spots for 10 minutes, then rinse.
● **For dry skin:** mix some turmeric powder with bio yogurt to make a paste. Apply to spots for 10 minutes, then rinse.

38 *Sardines*

Oily fish such as sardines are a rich source of long-chain omega-3 fatty acids (EPA and DHA), which have a powerful anti-inflammatory action to help damp down conditions like dandruff, acne and rosacea, and skin rashes such as eczema and psoriasis.

The flexible molecules in EPA and DHA are also incorporated into skin cell membranes to improve their softness, suppleness and ability to retain moisture. They also have a blood-thinning effect to boost circulation to hair, skin and nails, bringing in more oxygen and nutrients to promote healthy growth.

On the inside

As well as providing beneficial oils, sardines and other oily fish provide protein building

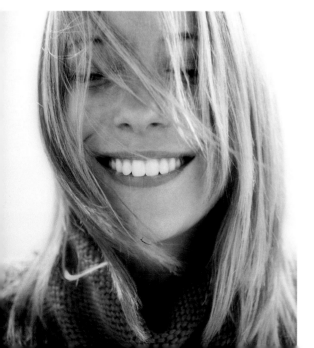

blocks for replenishing collagen, the main supporting structure of the skin, to help guard against fine lines and wrinkles. A steady supply of protein is also needed for the growth of strong, healthy hair and nails.

Combat skin ageing Omega-3 fish oils suppress the inflammatory responses that occur when skin is exposed to sunlight, and which lead to collagen degradation and wrinkles. A study involving more than 400 elderly people living in Greece, Australia and Sweden concluded that those with good intakes of tinned sardines showed 34 per cent fewer signs of skin ageing than those with low intakes.

Boost hair health Omega-3s help to combat dry, brittle hair and nails, hair loss and dry, flaky scalp. They boost hair strength, growth rate and gloss, as well as helping to overcome thinning hair.

Get a good smile Omega-3s help to reduce gum inflammation, associated with bad breath, receding gums and loss of teeth.

Omega-3s help to reduce gum inflammation.

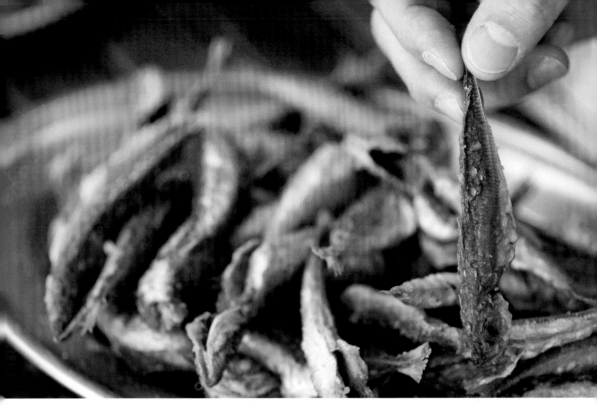

In your diet Aim to eat oily fish such as sardines, salmon, mackerel, trout, pilchards or herring at least once or twice a week. (NOTE: Girls and women of child-bearing age should eat no more than two portions a week, to reduce exposure to marine pollutants such as mercury, dioxins and polychlorinated biphenyls (PCBs), which can build up in the body and may affect future foetal development. Males, and women past reproductive age, can eat up to four portions of oily fish per week.)

On the outside

Deodorized fish oils are included in many cosmetic creams and hair products for their beneficial effects.

Beauty secrets
● For an instant glow, rather than swallowing a deodorized omega-3 fish oil capsule, pierce it and massage the fish oil directly onto your skin.

ALTERNATIVE SUPPLEMENTS

If you're not keen on eating more fish, take omega-3 fish oil capsules instead. If you are vegetarian, or allergic to fish, algae-derived DHA supplements are available instead; algae are at the bottom of the marine food chain, and are the ultimate source of much of the DHA present in fish oils.

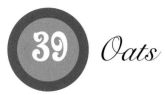

39 *Oats*

Rolled, flaked or ground to make oatmeal or flour, oats contain more protein than most other cereals and are an excellent source of B-group vitamins, which are vital for rapidly dividing cells in your hair, skin and nails.

On the inside

In addition to B vitamins, oats also supply important minerals (especially calcium and iron) and trace elements such as selenium. Eating oats helps to protect the skin from UV damage, partly due to the selenium content and partly due to the presence of an antioxidant amino acid called ergothioneine (EGT). EGT is unable to pass through the membrane of most body cells, but skin cells have recently been found to express a special EGT receptor. This allows EGT to accumulate in the skin, where it provides protection against the damaging effects of UV light, reducing the resulting level of sunburn and cell death.

In your diet Mainly eaten as porridge, muesli or granola, or in other types of cereal, this breakfast staple also tastes great in multigrain breads, oatcakes and cereal bars, and can even be added to fruit smoothies.

On the outside

Oats have been used since at least 2000 BCE to cleanse, soothe and beautify skin, and the Ancient Greeks, Romans and Egyptians added oats to baths to heal skin rashes. Oats contain unique antioxidants called avenanthramides, which soothe itchy, dry and irritated skin, and are gentle enough to add to baby skincare products, hair and bath products, and for use in sun-care products. Oatmeal is also great for acne-prone skin, because it absorbs oil from the skin's surface.

EGT derived from oats is added to many modern anti-ageing creams and cosmetics. Oat extracts are also added to some soothing eczema creams and bath soaks, and to shampoos and conditioners to help cleanse and soften hair and to reduce dandruff.

Eating oats helps to protect skin from UV damage.

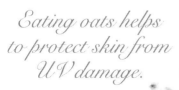

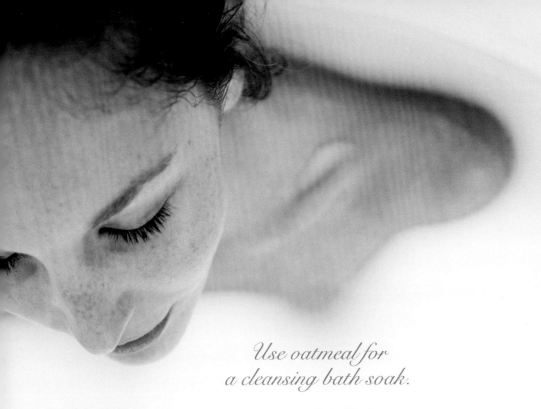

*Use oatmeal for
a cleansing bath soak.*

Beauty secrets

- **To exfoliate skin,** combine 2 tablespoons of live, natural bio yogurt (unsweetened) with 1 tablespoon of oats. Gently massage your skin with the mixture using a circular motion. (If your skin is dry, add 1 tablespoon of honey.)
- **To treat acne,** boil some oatmeal in water until it softens. Allow to cool for 15 minutes, then apply as a hot pack to the affected area, to absorb excess oil and exfoliate dead skin cells. Rinse after 10 minutes.
- **To relieve an itchy rash,** mix ground oatmeal with warm water to form a thick paste to apply to the area. Leave on for 10 minutes, then rinse. You can also add a handful of ground oatmeal to your bath water.
- **For a quick shampoo,** ground oats can be used as a dry shampoo for blond hair. Simply sprinkle some ground oats over your scalp to absorb oils, and brush out with a natural bristle brush.

 Top tip

For a cleansing bath soak, place oatmeal in a muslin bag/ cheesecloth and tie it to your bath tap so the water passes through when filling your bath. Squeeze periodically to release the milky water. You can also pat the wet pouch directly onto itchy skin.

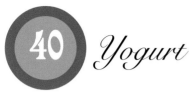

40 Yogurt

Live bio yogurt is a source of beneficial bacteria known as 'probiotics', the actions of which help to reduce bloating and discourage inflammatory conditions such as acne, rosacea and eczema. Yogurt also has an anti-ageing effect on skin.

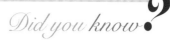

Did you know?

Other probiotic sources include sauerkraut, tempeh (fermented soy beans), miso, fermented dairy drinks, plus tablets, capsules and powders containing freeze-dried probiotic bacteria.

On the inside

Live bio yogurt is a dairy culture produced when beneficial, lactic-acid-producing bacteria ferment milk. Because these bacteria (probiotics) are acid-tolerant, a significant number survive passage through the stomach to reach the large intestines, where they discourage the growth of gas-forming bacteria and stimulate immunity, combating inflammatory conditions – but only if you eat the live, natural, *unsweetened* versions. Eating yogurt

Yogurt helps to combat signs of skin ageing.

with added sugar has been linked with an increased risk of acne.

Yogurt also appears to have an anti-ageing action on skin, and has been credited with contributing to the longevity of mountain populations in Bulgaria. Research comparing dietary intake with degree of skin wrinkling in volunteers aged seventy and over has also found that those with a good intake of yogurt showed 14 per cent fewer signs of skin ageing than those with low intakes.

Recommended dose If taking a probiotic supplement, select one containing a known quantity of live probiotic bacteria, such as 1–5 billion colony-forming units (CFU) per dose. Supplements that are enteric coated (which improves the survival of probiotic bacteria as they pass through the stomach) may contain fewer bacteria, but still provide beneficial effects.

Buying tip

Check the shelf life when buying probiotic supplements: those close to their expiry date contain fewer live probiotic bacteria than those with a longer shelf life.

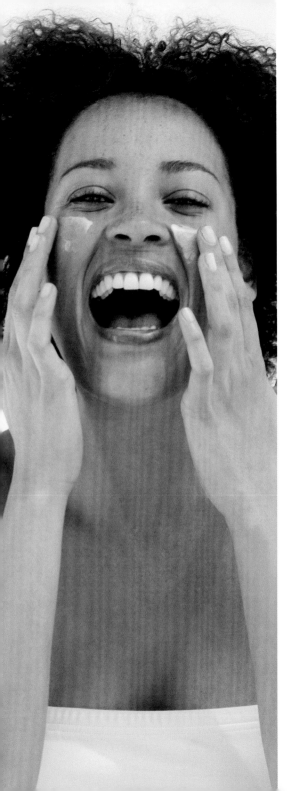

On the outside

Yogurt has been used since the time of Ancient Egypt for its beauty benefits to hair and skin. Cleopatra was known to take yogurt baths to help keep her skin soft, supple and youthful. As well as providing healthy bacteria to discourage those that cause blemishes, yogurt contains zinc and lactic acid to promote healthy skin. Yogurt facials help to remove dead skin cells, smooth fine lines, tighten pores, combat dryness and promote a healthy glow.

Beauty secrets

● **For silky, soft skin** split open a probiotic capsule and mix into 50 ml ($1^3/_4$ fl oz) natural, unsweetened Greek yogurt. Apply to your face, leave for 10 minutes, then rinse. Yogurt alone is also beneficial for discouraging spots and reviving a dull, tired complexion.

● **To treat dry skin** add 1 tablespoon of your favourite beauty oil (such as avocado, coconut, rosehip or evening primrose oil) to 4 tablespoons of thick bio yogurt. Apply to skin and leave for 15–30 minutes before rinsing.

● **To treat blackheads or whiteheads,** combine natural, unsweetened Greek yogurt with some rice powder to make a thick, coarse paste. Massage over the affected area, then rinse.

● **To even out skin tone and patchiness,** blend freshly squeezed lemon juice into thick bio yogurt, apply to your face and leave for 30 minutes before rinsing. (The acids in natural bio yogurt have a mild bleaching action, so yogurt alone will help to even out skin tone with regular use; combining with lemon juice simply provides a stronger effect.)

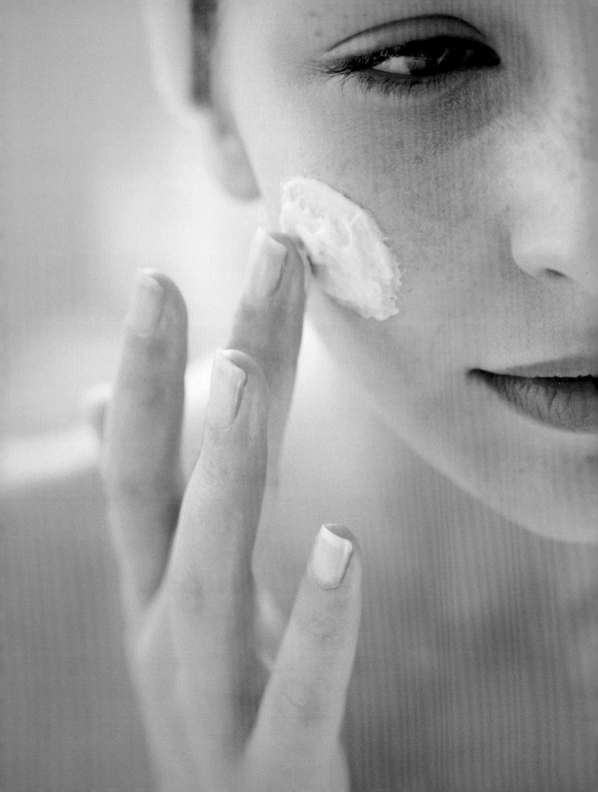

2

Beauty Clinic

What to eat – and what to avoid – to alleviate and prevent
over thirty common beauty problems, plus lifestyle checklists and
guidance on useful supplements and effective
salon techniques.

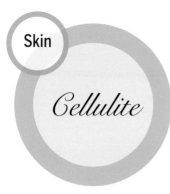

Cellulite

What causes it? Cellulite is linked with: female hormones • heredity • lack of exercise • high carbohydrate intake

Ask any woman about cellulite and she will know exactly what you mean. Three out of four could even show you some. But what can be done to prevent it?

➤➤ Cellulite – known medically as hydrolipodystrophy – is the name for dimpled skin in certain fat-storage areas of the body. It develops when fat cells in the hips, thighs or buttocks become overloaded. Islands of swollen cells bulge outwards and protrude into the lower skin layer (dermis), where they become squashed by the strands of fibrous connective tissue binding the skin together, to produce the typical, dimpled effect that resembles orange peel. Blood and lymph vessels running alongside these strands are slowly compressed as fat accumulates, to reduce the supply of oxygen and nutrients to affected tissues. As a result of poor blood circulation, cell wastes start to build up and affected areas may feel cold to touch.

Cellulite contains a higher than normal concentration of sugar-protein molecules known as glycosaminoglycans. These have moisture-attracting properties and can bind up to ten times their own weight of water. Tissues become waterlogged, soggy and sometimes tender. Unfortunately, the body responds to fluid accumulation and the build-up of waste products by laying down increasing amounts of fibrous tissue, which compresses the area further and makes the problem worse. Over a period of several years, the cell membranes of undernourished, swollen fat cells harden. This gives established cellulite its characteristic waxy, gritty, lumpy feel.

Lifestyle checklist

- Try Dead Sea mineral salts (used by Cleopatra and the Queen of Sheba as a beauty treatment): massage into the skin when bathing to stimulate circulation and exfoliate.
- Lose excess weight gradually: steady weight loss through diet and exercise will reduce subcutaneous collections of fat (avoid crash diets).
- Exercise daily for at least 30 minutes. Cycling, step aerobics, aerobics, light weights, walking and swimming are all excellent for toning up muscles and improving circulation.

Foods that can help

- **Follow a low-fat, wholefood diet** that is as organic as possible (some agricultural chemicals have an oestrogen-like action that may contribute to cellulite formation, although this is controversial).
- **Opt for a largely plant-based diet,** as animal-based foods contain hormones that may affect cellulite development.
- **Select wholegrain carbohydrate sources** such as brown rice and pasta, wholemeal bread, pulses and beans.
- **Eat oily fish regularly** (preferably organic): omega-3 fish oils have a beneficial effect on the circulation and the suppleness of cell membranes.

Omega-3 fish oils benefit circulation.

SALON TECHNIQUE

- **Ultrasound therapy** uses sound waves to break down and disperse cellulite – like being massaged from the inside out
- **Electro-muscular stimulation (EMS)** transmits a low-frequency impulse that stimulates muscles and dilates blood and lymphatic vessels
- **Vacuotherapy** applies negative suction to areas of cellulite to improve circulation, stimulate fat release, increase lymphatic drainage and ease the tethering of fibres that makes cellulite worse
- **Mesotherapy** involves a series of micro-injections into affected areas: tiny amounts of drugs and local anaesthetic are used to dilate small blood vessels, relax muscles, and stimulate blood and lymph circulation to help break down cellulite

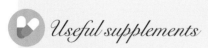

Useful supplements

Ginkgo biloba helps to open up circulation through small peripheral blood vessels and may improve blood flow in affected areas

Red vine leaf and **pine bark extracts** (Pycnogenol) strengthen supporting tissues to help reduce the spongy, dimpled appearance of cellulite

Gotu kola (*Centella asiatica*) is traditionally used to strengthen connective tissues; in trials, around 80 per cent of those taking this medicinal herb for three months reported 'satisfactory' to 'very good' results

Lecithin has a beneficial effect on the structure of fats, lowering cholesterol in the blood, and may have a beneficial effect on cellulite

Chromium may improve blood glucose regulation and reduce the conversion of sugar to fat

- **Use healthy oils** (such as flaxseed, pumpkin, walnut, olive, avocado, rapeseed) for cooking and in salad dressings.
- **Eat raw green vegetables** – raw greens are packed with fibre, antioxidants and enzymes that are said to have a cleansing effect on the bowel and help to remove toxins (eating them raw preserves more nutrients).
- **Drink water, herbal teas and fruit and vegetable juices** (unsweetened and diluted) to aid the elimination of toxins.

Foods to avoid

- **Cut back on carbohydrates** (especially sugars and refined flour) to follow a low-GI diet. This will reduce your secretion of insulin, which is the main fat-storing hormone in the body. A lower-carbohydrate diet is also associated with less fluid retention, as insulin affects the kidneys to reduce salt excretion. This means avoiding sugary foods and other refined carbohydrates (white flour products, cakes, biscuits, and so on).
- **Reduce salt intake** – select low-salt products and don't add salt during cooking or at the table.
- **Avoid saturated and trans fats** (found in margarines, for example) and processed meats (such as sausages and burgers).
- **Avoid artificial sweeteners**. It has been claimed that consuming artificial sweeteners is associated with cellulite; although there is no scientific evidence to support this, cutting them out will undoubtedly make your diet more healthy. Use stevia as a natural sweetener while you cultivate a taste for less-sweet foods.

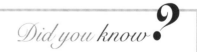

Did you know?

Cellulite is almost exclusively a feminine phenomenon. The female hormone, oestrogen, is thought to play a role, as it regulates the storage of body fat around the hips, thighs, bottom and knees.

Spinach, pomegranate, avocado & walnut salad

300 g (10 oz) baby spinach
leaves, rinsed and drained

¼ red onion, thinly sliced

1 ripe avocado, peeled and sliced

handful of walnut pieces

seeds from 1 pomegranate

FOR THE DRESSING:

1 tbsp lemon juice

2 tbsp walnut oil

1 clove garlic, crushed

freshly ground black pepper

Place all the salad ingredients in a bowl. Shake the dressing ingredients
together in a screw-top jar, then drizzle over the salad and serve.

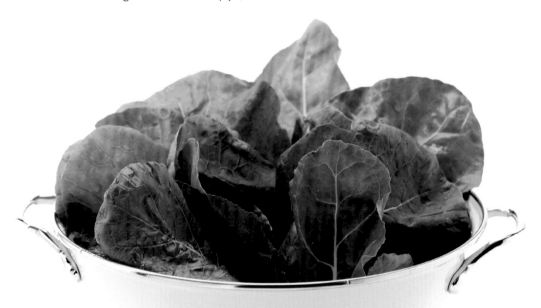

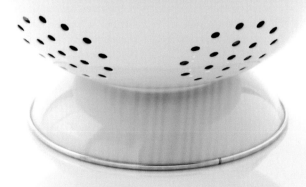

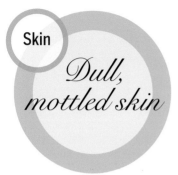

Skin

Dull, mottled skin

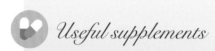

What causes it? Dull, mottled skin is linked with: age • vitamin and mineral deficiencies • low intake of carotenoid pigments found in fruit and vegetables

As skin ages, cell turnover slows, so it takes longer for new cells to reach the surface. Cells also stay on the surface for longer, meaning your skin may seem more dull and flaky than before. So what can you do to regain your youthful complexion?

➧➧ Your skin is one of the most nutritionally vulnerable parts of your body. The production of new skin cells requires good supplies of nutrients, and deficiency can affect skin quality at any age. During youth, it takes around one month for a newly formed skin cell to move from the lowest level of the skin to the surface. These cells are then shed and replaced with new skin cells, but as we get older, this process becomes slower.

Foods that can help

- **Eat plenty of fruit and veg:** the plant pigments they contain give your skin a healthy, slightly golden glow. Researchers at York, St Andrews and Cambridge

Useful supplements

Soy isoflavones help to boost oestrogen levels as the menopause approaches (recommended dose: 40–100 mg daily)

Probiotic supplements taken daily increase the conversion of soy isoflavones to a stronger form known as equol

universities in the UK have found that eating just two extra portions a day made a positive difference to skin tone as well as offering some protection against sunburn. The carotenoid pigments that are most beneficial are found in carrots, pumpkins, papaya, mango, sweet potato, bell peppers and dark green leafy vegetables (hidden by the green chlorophyll).
- **Say yes to soy:** plant isoflavones found in edamame beans and other soy products help to improve skin tone.
- **Drink green tea,** as it's a rich source of antioxidants that help to improve skin glow.

Lifestyle checklist

- Use SPF-based skincare creams and make-up providing a sun protection factor strength of at least SPF15.
- Use a good foundation providing high coverage to hide dull, mottled skin.
- Exfoliate skin weekly.
- Exercise briskly every day for at least 30 to 60 minutes, to increase skin blood flow.

Foods to avoid

- Cut back on foods that trigger free radicals and promote inflammation, such as omega-6-rich polyunsaturated cooking oils (especially sunflower, safflower and corn oils), added sugars, refined grains (especially gluten-containing wheat, rye and barley), processed meats (such as salamis, cheap sausages and meat pies), alcohol and deep-fried foods, including snacks like crisps.

Increasing your intake of soy isoflavones as the menopause approaches can help improve skin tone.

SALON TECHNIQUES

A variety of facial techniques are available to improve dull, mottled skin, including massage and exfoliation, plus:

- **Microdermabrasion** – a skincare technique that uses tiny rough grains to buff away the surface layer of skin
- **Intense pulsed light treatment (IPL)** – a non-invasive and non-ablative treatment that uses high-intensity pulses of visible light to improve the appearance of skin

Green Goddess smoothie

2 handfuls frozen, shelled edamame beans

flesh of 1 mango (fresh or frozen chunks)

500 ml (17 fl oz) soy milk (or a soy/coconut milk mix for a more tropical taste)

4 kale leaves or a handful of baby spinach leaves

Place all the ingredients in a blender and whizz until smooth. Add ice or more soy milk to obtain your desired consistency.

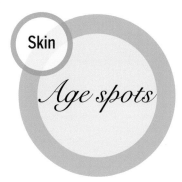

Skin

Age spots

What causes it? Age spots are linked with: sunbathing • sun beds • menopause and 'ageing'

Age spots are most often seen on the face, neck and backs of the hands and are related to previous sunburn. Help to keep them at bay by ensuring you get enough selenium in your diet – a vital mineral that protects against sun damage.

➡➡ Whenever your skin is exposed to the sun, ultraviolet rays generate free radicals. These set up an inflammatory reaction known as heliodermatitis, which leads to premature wrinkles and areas of hyperpigmentation commonly known as age spots (solar lentigo). Falling oestrogen levels at the menopause hasten the development of age spots, as the production of melanin pigment becomes less regulated without oestrogen.

Selenium provides important skin protection against sun damage, and low intakes increase the risk of developing age spots and certain types of skin cancer as much as sixfold. Selenium is so important for health that it's the only trace element whose incorporation into proteins is under direct genetic control. The selenoenzymes

Useful supplements

Selenium supplements are best taken in the form of selenium-enriched yeasts which increase the activity of antioxidant selenoenzymes more effectively than inorganic chemical sources such as selenium selenite

Co-enzyme Q10 helps cells absorb oxygen and produce energy; supplements have been shown to reduce some of the detrimental effects of photo-ageing

include a group of powerful antioxidants (glutathione peroxidases) which help to protect against UV-induced skin ageing.

Foods that can help
- **Step up the selenium:** the best food sources are Brazil nuts, fish, poultry, meats (especially game), wholegrains, mushrooms, onions, garlic, broccoli and cabbage, although the mineral content of crops depends on the soils in which they are grown and reared (in the USA and Canada, crops such as wheat are excellent sources, due to the levels of selenium present in the soil).

Lifestyle checklist
- Use sunscreen protection of at least SPF15 during both summer and winter months.
- Seek medical advice if an age spot or other skin lesion changes (for example, starts to get bigger, turn darker, go scaly, itch, weep, crust over or scab without healing, develop a raised, rolled edge or ulcerates).

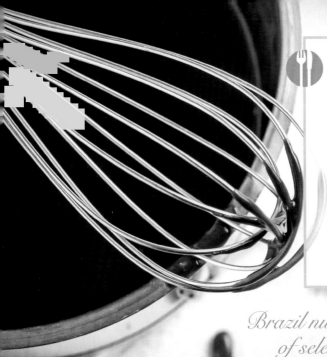

Dark chocolate Brazil nuts

150 g (5 oz) dark chocolate (at least 70 per cent cocoa solids)

50 whole, shelled Brazil nuts

Melt the chocolate in a bain-marie (heatproof bowl positioned over simmering water), then remove from the heat. Pour in the Brazil nuts and stir gently to coat fully. Remove each Brazil nut using a couple of teaspoons and place on greaseproof paper to set.

Brazil nuts are one of the best sources of selenium, which protects the skin against sun damage.

Top tip

Crushed guava leaves, papaya pulp, fresh strawberries, wheatgerm oil, pumpkin seed oil and rosehip oil can all be used topically to help fade age spots.

- **Increase your intake of antioxidants** by eating more fruit and veg – those found in pomegranates, papaya, berries, guava and watermelon are especially beneficial.
- **Plump for plant oestrogens** found in sweet potatoes, lentils, edamame beans and other soy products, to provide a useful oestrogen boost.

Foods to avoid
- **Steer clear of non-organic crops:** crops grown using sulphur-based fertilizers may have low selenium levels, as the chemicals affect selenium uptake by plants.

SALON TECHNIQUES
- **Medical treatments** of sun-damaged skin include tretinoin, a vitamin A derivative which helps to fade pigmented age spots and improve mottling
- **Over-the-counter fade creams** may include kinetin, a plant hormone derived from green leaves
- **Rosehip oil** applied daily to age spots has been found to produce significant improvements within three weeks, with brown hyperpigmentation almost completely fading within four months

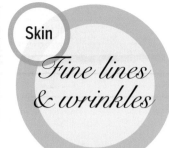

Skin
Fine lines & wrinkles

What causes it? Fine lines & wrinkles are linked with:
age • sun exposure • lack of oestrogen • smoking

Women's skin ages 25 per cent faster than men's between the ages of forty and fifty, due to the hormonal changes occurring around the menopause. Keep wrinkles at bay by getting plenty of protein and vitamin C in your diet.

➡ During your late twenties, fine lines (crinkles) and crow's feet develop around the eyes, where tissues are thin, delicate and easily stretched. During your thirties and forties, deeper, more extensive expression lines (linear furrows) appear. Skin cell renewal is now slowing and skin becomes drier. Brown age spots will develop on skin that has been exposed long-term to the sun.

When levels of oestrogen fall after the menopause, the production of collagen and elastin fibres slows, and those present become increasingly matted and tangled, so that skin loses its resilience and elasticity.

Lifestyle checklist

- Avoid excess sun exposure, don't use sun beds, and always wear sun protection products containing UVA and UVB sunscreens.
- Avoid smoking and limit your alcohol intake.
- Moisturize your skin well, both inside (fish oils, flaxseed and evening primrose oil) and out (argan, rosehip, avocado, macadamia and wheatgerm oils).
- Take regular exercise to boost skin circulation.
- Maintain good hydration.
- Avoid excess stress – cultivate laughter lines in place of frown lines!

Foods that can help

- **Eat plenty of protein:** lean protein provides building blocks to replenish collagen, the main supporting fibre in the skin. Women who eat a protein-rich diet (from eggs, skinless chicken, turkey, oily fish, lean beef, pulses, nuts and seeds) have fewer wrinkles and less skin fragility.
- **Bump up the vitamin C,** found in berries, pink grapefruit, pomegranate, mango, guava, green leaves and other fruits and vegetables. Vital for collagen production, it is also a powerful antioxidant, quenching the free radicals that promote wrinkles.
- **Choose carotenoids:** these yellow-orange plant pigments offer significant protection against sun damage and skin ageing.
- **Go green:** researchers have discovered that spinach and other green leafy vegetables offer the most protection of all vegetables against skin wrinkling.
- **Add a bit of spice:** turmeric and ginger reduce inflammation and help to prevent age-related tissue changes.

Did you know?

Smokers are five times more likely to develop premature wrinkles than non-smokers.

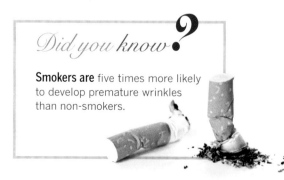

Useful supplements

Glucosamine provides building blocks for the formation of healthy connective tissue and improves the appearance of fine lines and wrinkles

Soy isoflavones protect skin against sun damage and reduce wrinkle formation in older women

Evening primrose oil supplements help moisturize skin from the inside

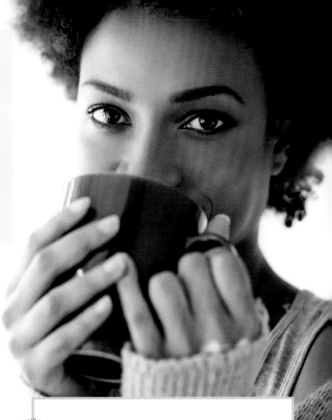

- **Enjoy a cuppa:** tea, especially green tea, contains powerful antioxidants, and those who drink a lot of tea have been found to have better skin and fewer wrinkles.
- **Get an oestrogen boost:** edamame beans, sweet potato and lentils are good sources of plant oestrogens that provide a useful boost for skin collagen production in later life.

Foods to avoid

- **Cut back on** polyunsaturated cooking oils (such as sunflower, safflower, corn), sugar, refined grains (especially wheat, rye and barley), processed meats (salamis, cheap sausages, meat pies), alcohol and deep-fried foods, including crisps.
- **Avoid processed foods that have been 'browned' by heat** (for example, toast, golden-brown chips, barbecued meat), as these contain appropriately named AGEs (advanced glycation end products) that damage cells, inhibit cellular renewal, trigger inflammation and hasten wrinkles.

SALON TECHNIQUES

- **Numerous options include** dermabrasion, fillers, Botox, platelet-rich plasma injections, suture suspension cones and surgical facelifts

Spinach, macadamia & pomegranate salad

1 bag baby spinach leaves, washed

1 small red onion, thinly sliced

handful of macadamia nuts

handful of beansprouts or edamame beans

seeds from 1 pomegranate

30 ml (1 fl oz) flaxseed, avocado or pumpkin seed oil

1 tsp balsamic vinegar

freshly ground black pepper

Toss all the ingredients together and serve immediately to accompany lean meat, fish or eggs for extra protein.

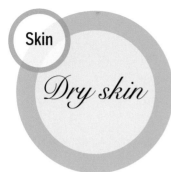

Dry skin

What causes it? Dry skin is linked with: heredity • over-exposure to water, harsh soaps, irritants or environmental conditions • lack of essential fatty acids • vitamin A deficiency

When the hydration level in our skin falls it starts to feel dry and itchy, and the normal process of skin cell shedding is reduced, causing cells to build up. Increasing your intake of omega-3s is just one of the ways you can help guard against this.

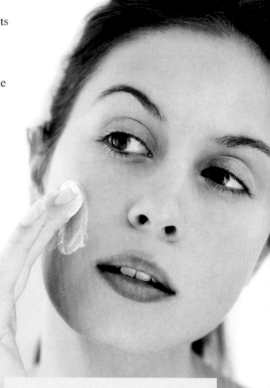

➤➤ The epidermis (outer layer of the skin) consists of approximately twenty layers of flattened, dead cells called corneocytes. These contain natural moisturizers that help to lock in water and retain a moisture level of around 30 per cent. By the time skin feels rough, dry and develops scaling, the water level of skin may be as low as 10 per cent.

Foods that can help

• **Boost your omega-3 intake.** Omega-3 essential fatty acids provide building blocks for making skin cell membranes that retain moisture more readily. They also suppress the inflammatory response that leads to itching and reduced skin cell shedding. Aim to eat oily fish like sardines, salmon, tuna,

Lifestyle checklist

• Apply an emollient moisturizer regularly, at least twice a day, including after bathing.
• Avoid soap, which is drying, and wash with an emollient cream instead.
• Avoid overly hot baths or showers, which trigger the release of histamine, making dry skin more itchy. Similarly, pat dry with a towel rather than rubbing.
• Use a bath or shower water filter that both removes chlorine and softens water (chlorine in water can irritate skin).
• Wear rubber gloves when washing dishes.

Useful supplements

Evening primrose oil provides essential fatty acids that moisturize skin when taken by mouth, producing significant improvements in scaliness and itching; it can also be applied directly onto patches of dry skin

mackerel or herring at least twice a week. Walnuts, flaxseeds, pumpkin seeds, chia and hemp are also good sources.
- **Eat more vitamin-C-rich foods** such as berries and mango: higher intakes are associated with better skin appearance due to improved collagen production and moisture retention.

Foods to avoid
- **Cut back on carbs** – lower intakes of carbohydrate are associated with improved skin appearance. Follow a low-GI (glycemic index) diet by avoiding refined grains such as white rice, white-flour breads, pasta and cakes, which raise insulin levels and promote inflammation.

SALON TECHNIQUES
- **Hydrotherapy** using silica-rich waters from the Avène dermatological spa in the South of France is used to treat dry skin conditions; water is available in spray bottles, and in a range of skincare products
- **Wheatgerm oil** is a particularly valuable treatment for dry skin, leaving it feeling soft and smooth

Warm sardines with mango & chickpea salad

400 g (14 oz) sardines in olive oil, drained (reserve oil)

1 large bag mixed green leaves

400 g (14 oz) can cooked chickpeas, drained

flesh from 1 mango, chopped

handful of flatleaf parsley, chopped

1 tsp balsamic vinegar

freshly ground black pepper

Preheat the oven or grill on a moderate setting. Place the sardines on an oven tray, brush with a little of the reserved oil and bake or grill for 5 minutes to warm through.

Toss the leaves, chickpeas, chopped mango and parsley in a bowl. Drizzle with the balsamic vinegar and a little of the reserved oil, season with black pepper, and serve with the warm sardines. Best enjoyed with wholegrain, crusty bread.

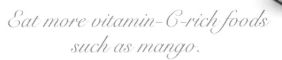

Eat more vitamin-C-rich foods such as mango.

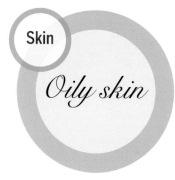

Skin

Oily skin

When the glands linked to hair follicles become overactive, oiliness and shine occur on the skin – most noticeably on the forehead, nose and chin. But you can help combat this through your diet ...

➤➤ Each of your hair follicles is linked to a sebaceous gland whose oily secretions (sebum) are designed to keep your hair sleek and waterproof. These follicles are found in the greatest number on your face and scalp, which is why oily skin becomes more apparent in these areas.

Foods that can help
- **Eat a diet rich in essential fatty acids** (EFAs), found in nuts, seeds and oily fish. If your skin is lacking in EFAs, it can become scaly and rough and lose water more easily. This drying out stimulates over-production of oil to compensate,

---

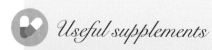

Useful supplements

Evening primrose oil is helpful if you have combination skin with dryness that leads to a compensatory increase in oil production

---

leading to so-called combination skin with a central oily patch and dry, itchy cheeks.
- **Increase your intake of lignans** – oestrogen-like hormones which inhibit 5-alpha reductase, an enzyme which stimulates increased oil production. Good sources are sweet potatoes and lentils; pumpkin seed oil also has a similar action.
- **Opt for avocado**: the monounsaturated fats found in avocado help to damp down any accompanying redness and inflammation.

Foods to avoid
- **Avoid sugary, stodgy foods**.
- **Cut back on cow's-milk products** to see if this helps (cow's milk increases insulin levels, which encourages the production of sebum). Try sheep's-, goat's- or soy-milk products instead, and be sure to eat plenty of wholegrains and dark green, leafy vegetables for calcium, to compensate.

Lifestyle checklist
- Select skincare products designed for your skin type – either oily or combination skin.
- Use a gentle exfoliative mask designed for your skin type.
- Opt for mineral-powder make-up, as it's more likely to stay in place without 'melting' or promoting increased oil production.
- Try a home-made face mask to reduce skin oiliness using bilberries, honey or turmeric (see pages 41, 73 and 81).

SALON TECHNIQUES

● **Argan oil** is commonly used by facialists to both moisturize dry skin areas and normalize excess oiliness; twice daily use for four weeks has been shown to significantly reduce skin greasiness

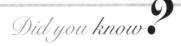

Did you know

If your skin is oily, the good news is that you are likely to develop wrinkles less quickly than those with dry skin – unless you smoke.

Sweet potato, lentil & coriander soup

3 tbsp avocado oil

1 tsp turmeric or curry powder

1 onion, chopped

2 cloves garlic, crushed

1 apple, peeled, cored and chopped

thumb-sized piece fresh ginger, grated

handful of coriander leaves/stalks, chopped

500 g (1 lb 2 oz) sweet potatoes, peeled and chopped

800 ml (1½ pt) vegetable stock

100 g (3½ oz) red lentils

200 ml (7 fl oz) soy milk

zest and juice of 1 lime

freshly ground black pepper and sea salt

Fry the turmeric/curry powder and onions in the avocado oil for 2 minutes. Add the garlic, apple, ginger and coriander leaves/stalks and fry gently for 5 minutes. Add the sweet potatoes, vegetable stock, lentils and soy milk and simmer gently for around 20 minutes until the potatoes are soft and the lentils are cooked. Blend until the lime zest/juice, season to taste, and serve garnished with a few coriander leaves.

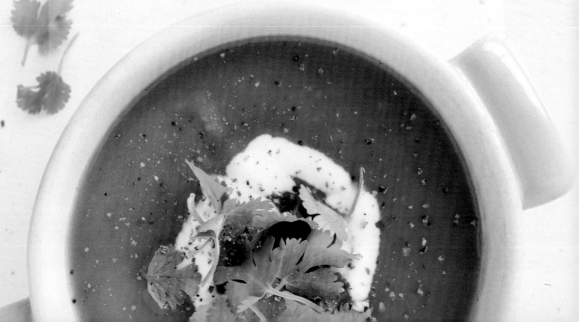

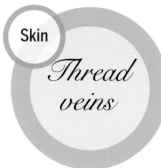

Thread veins

What causes it? Thread veins are linked with: exposure to extremes of temperature • lack of vitamin C • possibly lack of vitamin K • an inflammatory skin condition known as rosacea

Many of us suffer from visible, red, dilated blood vessels, especially on the cheeks and nose. Following an alkaline diet can help, as can ensuring that you consume plenty of vitamin K.

▶▶ Known as telangiectasia, these dilated blood vessels are believed to result from hypersensitivity of facial blood capillaries in the skin which do not constrict back down after dilation (for example, in response to heat or alcohol). Over time, they can increase in size, causing capillary walls to weaken. Thread veins can occur around hair follicles as an early sign of vitamin C deficiency.

Foods that can help

- **Bring on the bilberries:** bilberries are used to strengthen blood vessels and to improve circulation through tiny capillaries.
- **Try an alkaline diet:** some people find it helpful to follow an alkaline diet that avoids acid-forming foods. This means eating more fruit and vegetables, and cutting back on some grains (barley, oats, quinoa, rice, wheat), dairy products (cheese, milk, ice cream, yogurt), animal proteins (eggs, poultry, meats, seafood), beer and wine. However, these foods are important sources of protein, vitamins and minerals, so it is advisable to follow a strict alkaline diet under the supervision of a medical nutritionist.
- **Eat vitamin-K-rich foods,** such as green leafy vegetables, tomatoes, prunes, edamame beans, pumpkin seeds, wheatgerm oil and probiotic bacteria found in live yogurt.

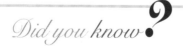

Useful supplements

Bilberry extracts (often prescribed in parts of Europe) benefit circulation and help strengthen the walls of blood vessels

Pine bark extracts (Pycnogenol) strengthen fragile capillaries and reduce abnormal blood clotting – even in smokers

Vitamin K$_2$ (more active than vitamin K$_1$) promotes a healthy cardiovascular system thanks to its ability to optimize calcium utilization

---

Did you know?

Vitamin K is involved in blood clotting and may help to seal leaking capillaries in those who are deficient. Vitamin K gel has been shown to improve the response to facial thread veins treated with a pulsed dye laser.

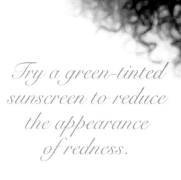

Try a green-tinted sunscreen to reduce the appearance of redness.

Lifestyle checklist

- Use a broad-spectrum, high-protection sunscreen or sunblock that protects against both UVA and UVB light.
- Try a green-tinted sunscreen to reduce the appearance of redness.
- Avoid applying astringents, toners or products containing sodium lauryl sulphate, which can irritate the skin.
- Avoid temperature extremes.
- Try gently rubbing a wedge of tomato on dilated veins.

Foods to avoid

- **Avoid consuming** spicy foods, coffee, tea, sodas, foods with preservatives, colourings, artificial sweeteners and other additives.

SALON TECHNIQUES

- **Creams or gels containing vitamin K** are used to treat skin redness and visible small capillaries
- **Intense pulsed light** (IPL) or **dye laser resurfacing** can improve dilated veins

Wilted spinach & tomatoes with pumpkin seeds

dash of olive oil

handful of pumpkin seeds

12 cherry tomatoes, halved

2 bags baby spinach leaves, washed

1 tbsp balsamic vinegar

freshly ground black pepper

pumpkin oil or wheatgerm oil (optional)

Heat the oil in a pan. Add the pumpkin seeds and tomatoes and cook, stirring, for a couple of minutes. Add the spinach and cook, tossing often, until just wilted. Stir in the vinegar and season to taste. Drizzle the final result with a little pumpkin oil or wheatgerm oil for additional vitamin K, if desired.

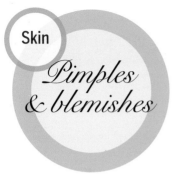

Skin

Pimples
& blemishes

What causes it? Pimples and blemishes are linked with: blockage of blackheads • overgrowth of the skin bacterium *Propionibacterium acnes*

Researchers are now finding increasing evidence that nutrition has a profound effect on skin health, so watching what you eat really can help to guard against the formation of spots and blemishes.

➡ We all get spots from time to time. In fact, your diet can influence the secretion of skin oil (sebum), the stickiness of skin cells (keratinocytes) and whether or not they are shed. If they clump together, they can block sebaceous gland ducts to trap oil and form blackheads (see also pages 108–9). Diet also influences whether or not the skin bacterium *P. acnes* flourishes on the skin, and the degree of inflammation that results.

Foods that can help

- **Eat more oily fish:** omega-3 fatty acids (especially DHA and EPA, found in oily fish such as sardines) have an anti-inflammatory action to help damp down inflamed skin.

- **Get your five-a-day:** fruit and vegetables provide vitamins, minerals and antioxidants that help to reduce inflammation.
- **Increase fibre intake:** a high-fibre diet helps to slow absorption of sugars and reduce blood-glucose swings and insulin secretion.
- **Plump for pumpkin:** pumpkin seed oil helps to reduce skin oiliness and spots.
- **Go for garlic** – it has a natural, antibacterial action.

Foods to avoid

- **Avoid a high-GI diet:** spots are linked with following a high glycemic diet that contains significant amounts of sugars

Lifestyle checklist

- Look for non-comedogenic skincare products, as these don't promote blackhead formation.
- Remove make-up scrupulously with a pH (acid)-balanced, non-perfumed cleanser.
- Avoid picking or squeezing spots, as this spreads bacteria, producing longer-lasting pimples that are more likely to scar.
- Drink guava or carrot juice (or use them in topical applications) – both popular remedies for spots.

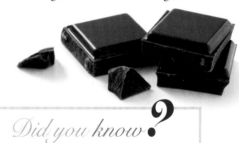

Did you know?

Despite chocolate's reputation for causing spots, dark chocolate containing at least 72 per cent cocoa solids may actually improve symptoms, as it's one of the richest dietary sources of anti-inflammatory antioxidants.

and refined carbohydrates. This rapid swing in blood glucose levels triggers the release of insulin and a related substance called insulin-like growth factor (IGF-1). These stimulate the growth and proliferation of skin cells, making them more sticky, so that they clump together rather than being shed, blocking oil gland ducts and causing blackheads.

- **Cut back on cow's milk:** milk contains sugars, growth factors and hormones that can affect the skin. Researchers have found that adolescents who consume more than two servings a day are more likely to have acne than those consuming fewer dairy products. If cutting back, ensure a good calcium intake from wholegrains and dark green, leafy vegetables. You could also try goat's milk/butter, and switching from milk chocolate to dark chocolate.

SALON TECHNIQUES
- **Treatments such as** suction dermabrasion, vacuum extraction, intense pulsed light and vascular lasers can help

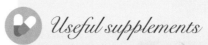

Useful supplements

Probiotic supplements may help (an abnormal balance of bowel bacteria may play a role in skin blemishes)

Vitamin C helps spots to heal

Vitamin A and betacarotene discourage dry, raised, pimply hair follicles

Zinc supplements have, in some cases, been proven as effective as antibiotics for treating spots (zinc deficiency can trigger spots)

Sardine, spinach & pumpkin salad

225 g (8 oz) sardines, tinned in olive or sardine oil

I bag baby spinach leaves, washed

4 slices of roast pumpkin, skinned and chopped

12 baby tomatoes, halved

1 small red onion, thinly sliced

½ cucumber, chopped

FOR THE DRESSING:
juice and zest of 1 unwaxed lemon

2 tbsp pumpkin seed oil

1 clove garlic, crushed

freshly ground black pepper

Place all the salad ingredients in a bowl. Put the dressing ingredients in a small screw-top jar and shake to combine, then drizzle over the salad.

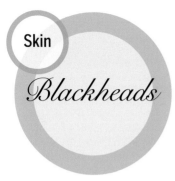

Blackheads

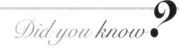

What causes it? **Blackheads are linked with:** genetics • hormone imbalances (especially at puberty) • oral contraceptives • some skincare products that clog pores

The tiny pores in your skin are the openings of your hair follicles. If these pores become clogged, blackheads may form, so reducing skin oiliness is key – and sweet potato may be the answer!

➥ Each hair follicle contains an oil gland that secretes greasy sebum to condition your growing hair. If you produce excessive amounts of thick oil, or if the skin pores become clogged with unshed skin cells, the oily secretions build up to form a blackhead, or comedo. Blackheads (comedones) are open pores; their frequent companions, whiteheads, are blocked pores where sebum is trapped just beneath the surface of the skin, without an obvious opening onto the skin surface. Bacteria can become trapped in blocked pores to cause an outbreak of spots.

Did you know?

The dingy colour of blackheads is due to dissolved, oxidized skin pigments (melanin) and dead skin cells rather than dirt, as is commonly believed.

Sweet potato & coconut mash

600 g (1 lb 5 oz) sweet potatoes
100 ml (3½ fl oz) coconut milk
1 tbsp freshly grated ginger
freshly ground black pepper and sea salt

Prick the sweet potatoes all over with a fork and microwave for 10–15 minutes (or bake in the oven for 1 hour) until tender. Scoop out the flesh with a spoon and discard the skins. Mash the sweet potato together with the coconut milk and ginger. Season to taste. Reheat and serve with sardines, salmon, tuna or cold meats and salad.

Foods that can help

- **Switch to sweet potato!** Over-production of skin oils – leading to clogged pores – can result from hormone imbalances or an increased sensitivity of oil glands to normal hormone levels. Foods such as sweet potatoes and lentils contain oestrogen-like lignans that suppress the production of dihydrotestosterone hormone (DHT) in hair follicles, to reduce skin oiliness and comedo formation.
- **Eat like a Kitavan:** native residents of an island called Kitava, near Papua New Guinea, eat a lot of sweet potato, fruit, seafood and coconuts, and are said not to develop blackheads or acne.

Foods to avoid

- **Try avoiding coffee, tea, alcohol and dairy products,** none of which are included in the native Kitavan diet (if cutting back on dairy, make sure you still

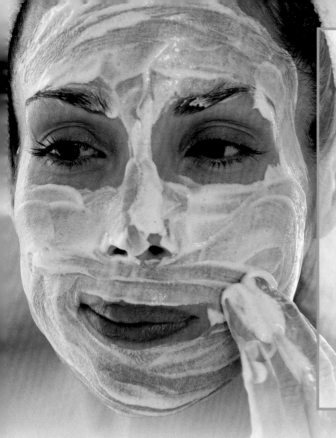

get plenty of calcium from green, leafy vegetables or plant-based milks).
- **Avoid high-GI foods:** the Kitavan diet is also low-GI, containing no added sugar apart from that obtained in fruit.

SALON TECHNIQUES
- **Pore-extracting strips** help to remove blackheads (though they will recur without a proper skincare regime)
- **Pumpkin seed oil** is used by facialists to gently 'dissolve' dry surface skin cells, reduce pore size and blackheads, and control excess oiliness
- **Microdermabrasion** and **'acid' peels** are used professionally to dissolve blackheads
- **Vitamin A derivatives** can be prescribed

to both treat and prevent blackheads; over-the-counter preparations containing retinol are also available

 Useful supplements

Vitamin C is an important antioxidant in skin to discourage infection

Omega-3 fish oil supplements are a useful alternative if you don't like eating fish

A multivitamin and mineral supplement that includes vitamin A will guard against deficiencies that can increase comedo formation

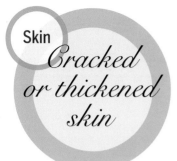

Skin
Cracked or thickened skin

What causes it? Cracked or thickened skin is linked with: age • rubbing and pressure from ill-fitting shoes • high heels • lack of essential fatty acids

If you walk an average of 5,000 steps a day, you will clock up over 80,000 miles during your lifetime – the equivalent of walking more than three times round the equator! So why not help save your soles through your diet ...

➡➡ While 5,000 steps a day may sound like a lot, the recommended advice for optimum health benefits is to walk *twice* that. But what effect does all this strolling have on our feet? A build-up of thick skin is common, and can lead to unsightly calluses (known as corns, when they form on your toes) and painful cracks on the heels that can make us reluctant to bare our feet in summer or wear flip-flops or sandals.

Useful supplements

Evening primrose oil and **omega-3 fish oils** help to moisturize skin from the inside

Supplements combining garlic, ginkgo and ginger improve peripheral blood flow

Lifestyle checklist
- Massage a few drops of argan, wheatgerm or coconut oil/coconut butter into cracked skin on heels and elbows. Avocado pulp is also a popular home treatment for cracked heels.
- Make a strawberry foot scrub to exfoliate dry skin by mashing together eight strawberries, 2 tablespoons of oil (such as argan, wheatgerm, coconut or olive oil) and 1 teaspoon of sea salt.
- Use a foot spa to soften skin and pamper aching feet. The latest home models combine magnetic therapy and rotating buffers along with a warm soak.
- Wear gel shoe insoles and pads to cushion painful areas.

Foods that can help
- **Spice things up:** eating spicy foods containing chilli, garlic and ginger for their natural warming action promotes the dilation of blood vessels to improve the delivery of blood, oxygen and vital nutrients to your feet.
- **Eat more oily fish:** omega-3 fish oils provide essential fatty acids, which reduce inflammation and, when incorporated into skin cell membranes, help make them more soft and supple thanks to their flexible structure.
- **Eat plant-based foods** – especially edamame and other soy products, sweet potato and lentils – as these provide natural anti-inflammatory phytosterols and phytoestrogens that improve skin quality.

- **Ensure good intakes of vitamin A, vitamin E and zinc:** vitamin A is formed from yellow-orange carotenoid pigments found in fruit, vegetables and green leaves, as well as pre-formed in animal-based foods; vitamin E is found in various foods, especially plant oils (wheatgerm oil is the richest natural source); and zinc is found in seafood, wholegrain cereals and red meat.

Foods to avoid

- **Don't overcook your veg!** This deactivates vitamins and leaches minerals and phytonutrients into the cooking water. Eat vegetables raw or only lightly steamed, where possible, and reclaim cooking water to make sauces, soups, gravies or dhal.

SALON TECHNIQUES

- **Professional pedicures** can buff away thickened skin, but see a chiropodist if you need skin physically cut away – never do this yourself!

Spicy, warming, lentil dhal soup

750 ml (1⅓ pt) vegetable or chicken stock, or water

200 g (7 oz) red lentils, rinsed

thumb-sized piece of fresh ginger, peeled and sliced

2 bay leaves

1 fresh chilli, sliced down the middle

1 cinnamon stick

30 ml (1 fl oz) olive oil (or ghee/clarified butter)

1 large onion, chopped

4 cloves garlic, crushed

2 tsp turmeric

1 tsp cumin

juice and zest of 1 lemon

handful of coriander leaves, chopped

freshly ground black pepper and sea salt

Simmer the lentils, ginger, bay leaves, chilli and cinnamon in the stock/water for 15 minutes, stirring regularly. Sauté the onion, garlic, turmeric and cumin in the oil (or ghee) for 5 minutes, add the lentil mixture along with the lemon juice and zest, and cook for a further 3 minutes, stirring constantly. Add the coriander leaves and season to taste.

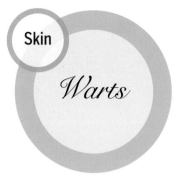

Skin

Warts

What causes it? Warts are linked with: human papilloma virus (HPV) • long-term sun exposure can cause lesions resembling warts

Caused by infection with a skin virus, common warts usually affect areas of skin prone to injury, such as the hands, elbows, face, knees and scalp. If left untreated, they usually clear within a year, though most of us would rather not wait that long ...

▶▶ In older people, long-term sun exposure can cause wart-like skin lesions known as actinic keratosis (AK), which, in some cases, can progress to form skin cancer. They are usually treated to prevent this happening. These take the form of rough, sandpapery patches of skin on sun-exposed areas that may be red, tan, pink or flesh-toned. They are often elevated to resemble warts. One in ten people over the age of forty has AK, rising to one in four people aged sixty or over. Seek medical advice if you think you might have one. Treatment includes medicated creams or gels to 'melt' them away, cryotherapy to freeze and shrink them, or laser surgery to burn them off.

Warts on the soles of the feet become flattened by the weight of the body to form painful verrucas (plantar warts).

Lifestyle checklist

- **Don't scratch!** Never squeeze or scratch warts, or the virus may spread; scratching also increases the chance of scarring.
- **Try duct tape:** home remedies include applying duct tape (said to work due to ingredients in its adhesive). Leave the tape on for three days, remove it and file off the dead skin, repeating until the wart is gone. Another popular home remedy is to dab the wart regularly with tea tree essential oil.
- **Be mindful of others:** warts are contagious and can be passed on through direct contact (although many people are naturally immune).
- **Seek medical advice** if you think you might have actinic keratosis, or if a wart, beauty mark or other skin lesion changes in any way (enlarges, darkens, itches, bleeds, and so on).
- **Never treat genital warts yourself** – visit a sexual health clinic.

BEAUTY SPOTS

These dark facial moles (known medically as melanocytic nevus) are caused by a developmental clustering of pigment cells and, unlike warts, do not disappear spontaneously. They may be present from birth, or may develop up to the age of around thirty. Though generally considered attractive, if you do wish to have one removed, consult an aesthetic dermatologist – do not try to treat it yourself.

Foods that can help

- **Reach for the garlic:** garlic has a natural antiviral action, and eating it daily may help a common wart to clear. (Applying fresh garlic juice is a popular home remedy, but be sure to protect the surrounding skin with petroleum jelly, as this treatment can cause blistering.)

- **Anti-wart treatments** are widely available from pharmacies; warts can be frozen off professionally, or using home wart-freezing kits

Useful supplements

Grapefruit seed extracts (available as liquid) may be applied undiluted to a common wart (apply one drop, twice daily)

Garlic sauce

cloves from 1 garlic bulb, peeled and crushed

100 ml (3½ fl oz) fresh lemon juice

200 ml (7 fl oz) olive oil
(not extra virgin)

1 tsp sea salt

Place all the ingredients in a blender and whizz until the mixture thickens to the texture of mayonnaise. Serve with grilled fish, meats or as a salad dressing.

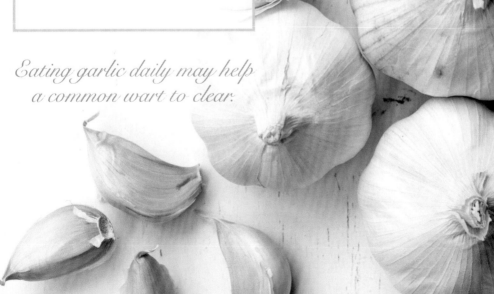

Eating garlic daily may help a common wart to clear.

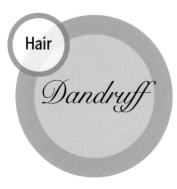

Dandruff

What causes it? Dandruff is linked with: pityrosporum yeasts • lack of essential fatty acids • lack of vitamins A, B₂, B₃, B₆, C, biotin and the minerals iodine, manganese, selenium and zinc • stress (neurodermatitis) • shampoo allergy

This annoying build-up of unsightly white flakes on the scalp and in the hair occurs when dead cells clump together to form larger, visible flakes. But there are plenty of ways you can combat this common problem through your diet.

Skin on the scalp is continually replaced, just like skin elsewhere on the body. Dead cells that fall off are usually washed or brushed away, but if the cells are replaced faster than normal, or if the scalp is excessively dry or greasy, dead cells may clump together to form larger, visible flakes.

Simple dandruff with flakiness but no redness or inflammation is known as pityriasis capitis. More severe dandruff, associated with inflammation, redness, itching and dry or greasy scales, is known as seborrhoeic dermatitis.

Foods that can help

- **Increase intake of EFAs:** dandruff is sometimes linked with lack of essential fatty acids, so aim to eat more oily fish such as sardines, nuts, seeds and wholegrains. Eating a handful of macadamia nuts per day significantly improves inflammation, and omega-3 essential fatty acids (found in oily fish and flaxseed, for example) also help by reducing inflammation.

- **Get your vital vitamins!** Dry, scaly skin has been linked with lack of vitamins A (found in animal products, and formed

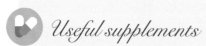

Useful supplements

Evening primrose, flaxseed and **omega-3 fish oils** provide essential fatty acids

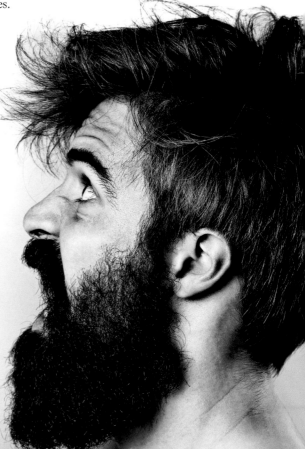

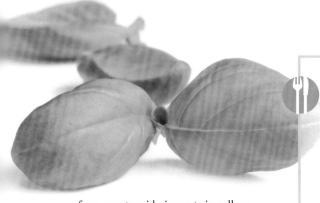

from carotenoid pigments in yellow-orange fruit and vegetables), B₂ and B₃ (found in wholegrains, green leafy vegetables and beans), C (found in berries, guava, pink grapefruit), biotin (oily fish, wholegrains, nuts), and the minerals iodine (marine fish, seaweed), manganese (green tea and other green leaves), selenium (Brazil nuts) and zinc (seafood, meat, wholegrains). In addition, vitamin B_6 helps prevent dandruff and is found in cereals, egg yolk and liver.

Foods to avoid

- **Cut back on processed foods and margarines,** which provide omega-6 fatty acids that promote inflammation.
- **Cut back on excess sugar** and follow a low-glycemic diet.
- **Avoid cow's milk products for two weeks,** to see if this reduces inflammation (ensure you obtain calcium from other sources such as wholegrains, broccoli and dark green leaves).

SALON TECHNIQUES

- **Hair salons** can advise on professional haircare products designed to minimize dandruff. If there is no improvement after two weeks of using an anti-fungal shampoo (containing ketoconazole or selenium), seek medical advice, as stronger treatments are available on prescription

Macadamia nut pesto

1 bunch fresh basil leaves

60 ml (2 fl oz) Greek style soy- or sheep's-milk yogurta

2 handfuls roasted macadamia nuts

60 g (2 oz) Parmesan cheese, grated

juice of 1 lemon

salt and freshly ground black pepper

Put all the ingredients in a food processor and blend to your desired consistency – smooth or nutty. Delicious served cold as a dip with crudités, or warm served with wholegrain pasta.

Lifestyle checklist

- Rinse with diluted, unsweetened cranberry juice after shampooing (dilute 1:1 with water) to enhance colour and shine of red-brown hair and reduce dandruff.
- Apply tomato pulp to your scalp for 30 minutes before shampooing, to loosen stubborn, clinging flakes.
- Loosen scalp scales by gently rubbing with a tablespoon of argan, coconut, flaxseed or guava seed oil before shampooing. This soothes dry, sensitive skin and helps to damp down inflammation. If leaving on overnight, wear a shower cap or turban to protect your pillowcase. After a few treatments, most seborrhoeic scales should have gone.
- Use a clean, soft-bristled hairbrush to avoid transferring pityrosporum yeasts.

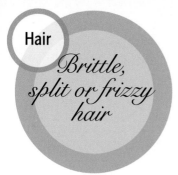

Hair

Brittle, split or frizzy hair

What causes it? Brittle, split or frizzy hair is linked with: genetics • lack of essential fatty acids • deficiency of vitamins A, C and minerals, especially iron, zinc or iodine • age • menopause • underactive thyroid gland

Nutritional deficiencies can lead to hair that is dry, frizzy or brittle with split ends. Eating more legumes can help! These contain one of the key nutrients required for good hair health.

▶▶ During your twenties, your hair is usually healthy, shiny and soft. New hair is constantly growing through, and you have between 100,000 and 150,000 active hair follicles on your scalp. As hair follicle cells are constantly dividing, they need a consistent supply of protein, vitamins and minerals – so it's up to us to make sure they get the fuel they need.

Vitamin A has a direct action on the nucleus of cells within hair follicles to strengthen hair shafts and reduce brittleness. Vitamin B_5 (pantothenic acid) also gives hair flexibility, strength and shine. Vitamin C is essential for the production of collagen protein, which is found in hair follicles, and,

together with keratin, is important for hair strength. Folic acid also contributes to follicle cell division and hair growth. Research from Harvard University suggests that biotin is one of the most important nutrients for preserving hair strength and texture.

Foods that can help

● **Eat the right vitamins and minerals.** Vitamin A is found in animal proteins such as eggs, meat and liver, and can be formed from yellow-orange carotenoid pigments found in fruit and vegetables such as carrots, dark green leaves (also an important source of folate – the natural form of folic acid – and iron) and sweet

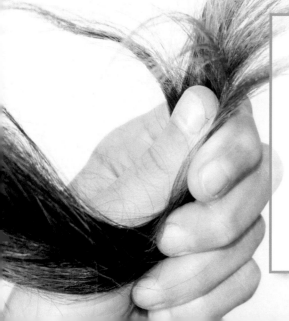

Lifestyle checklist

● Avoid using heat when drying or styling hair. Heat stretches and breaks the relatively weak hydrogen bonds in hair.
● Wrap your hair in a turban to absorb excess water after shampooing, then leave uncovered to dry naturally.
● Apply argan, rosehip, macadamia or coconut oil to hair to condition dry, brittle strands (applying argan oil after washing locks in moisture and shortens drying time).
● Trim hair regularly to remove split ends.

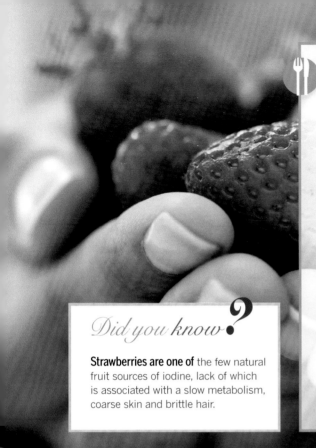

Strawberry, carrot & lentil salad

1 bag mixed green leaves

250 g (9 oz) cooked red lentils

2 carrots, peeled and grated

1 small red onion, finely chopped

handful of parsley leaves, chopped

16 strawberries, halved

FOR THE DRESSING:
2 tbsp flaxseed, pumpkin seed, avocado or olive oil

zest and juice of 1 lemon

1 clove garlic, crushed

freshly ground black pepper

Place the mixed green leaves in a bowl. Combine the remaining salad ingredients and pile on top of the leaves. Place the dressing ingredients in a small screw-top jar and shake to mix. Season to taste, and drizzle over the salad.

Did you know?

Strawberries are one of the few natural fruit sources of iodine, lack of which is associated with a slow metabolism, coarse skin and brittle hair.

potatoes. Vitamin C is found in most fruit and veg, especially berries, citrus fruits, bell peppers, tomatoes, mango, papaya and guava.

- **Increase your omega-3s:** omega-3 fatty acids, found in oily fish and flaxseed oil, are needed to strengthen hair and provide flexibility and moisture retention.
- **Love those legumes!** Legumes such as soy beans and lentils provide protein, iron, zinc and the key nutrient, biotin.

SALON TECHNIQUES

● **Intensive conditioner treatments** are offered by most hair salons (check the price, as they can be expensive)

 ### *Useful supplements*

A multivitamin and mineral supplement will guard against nutritional deficiencies

Evening primrose, flaxseed and **omega-3 fish oils** provide essential fatty acids

MSM (methylsulphonylmethane) boosts production of collagen and keratin protein

Biotin is worth trying, especially if you also have brittle nails

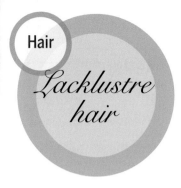

Lacklustre hair

What causes it? Lacklustre hair is linked with: lack of essential fatty acids, iron and vitamins E, B₅ and B₁₂ • over-use of heat • damage from hairbrushes and combs

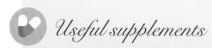

The outer layer of each hair (the cuticle) consists of thousands of tiny scales that overlap each other to form a smooth, light-reflecting surface. When these scales are smoothly aligned, hair has a healthy shine, but if they're ruffled or damaged, then hair becomes dull.

➡ Hair is a protein filament produced within hair follicles. During active growth, the root is tightly surrounded by live tissue called the hair bulb, which contains a layer of dividing cells. As new cells are formed, older ones die and are pushed upwards to form the extending hair shaft. Each hair shaft has a spongy central medulla containing air spaces, a middle cortex containing flexible chains of amino acids, and an outer hair cuticle, the condition of which dictates how our hair looks.

Foods that can help
- **Eat more oily fish,** such as salmon, mackerel and sardines: these provide

Mapled macadamias

250 g (9 oz) shelled macadamia nuts

1 tbsp macadamia nut oil (or olive oil)

1 tbsp maple syrup or honey

freshly ground black pepper (optional)

Preheat the oven to 180°C/350°F/Gas Mark 4. Toss the nuts in a bowl with the oil and maple syrup/honey to coat. Pour onto a baking tray and bake for 10 minutes. Season with black pepper if desired – but don't add salt!

Useful supplements

Omega-3 fish oils improve hair texture and shine

Royal jelly is one of the richest sources of vitamin B₅

omega-3 fatty acids, protein, vitamin B₁₂ and iron – all important for healthy, gleaming hair (deficiency can result in a dry scalp and dull hair). Vegetarian sources of omega-3 fats include ground flaxseed, macadamia nuts and walnuts.
- **Boost your B₅:** vitamin B₅ (pantothenic acid) gives hair flexibility, strength and shine and is found in wholegrains, beans, green leafy vegetables, nuts, eggs, meats and yeast extract.
- **Drink pomegranate juice** – this is said to improve hair lustre.

Foods to avoid
- **Don't add salt!** – either during cooking or at the table. Salt has a dehydrating effect on hair to reduce shine and increase hair thinning.

SALON TECHNIQUES
- **Intensive conditioner treatments** are offered by most hair salons to smooth

hair and add shine (check the price, as they can be expensive)

● **Hi-tech hairbrushes** are now available, including ones impregnated with argan oil or with tourmaline gem tips to revitalize hair and add shine

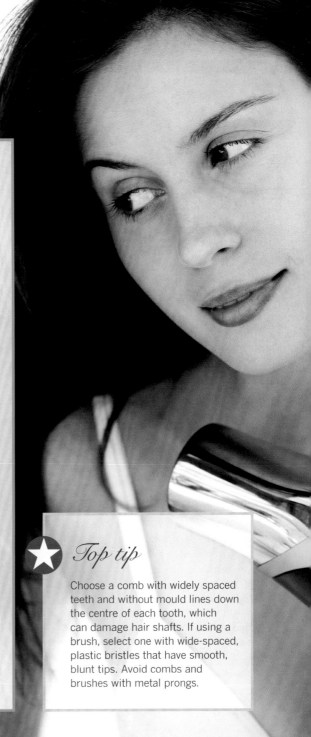

Lifestyle checklist

● Remove tangles before and after washing using a wide-toothed comb, working on the ends first, then gradually detangling further up the shaft towards the roots.
● Use a conditioner after shampooing to detangle and smooth hair shafts: fine, limp hair needs body-building products; curly, frizzy or chemically treated hair needs more intensive moisturizing. Apply conditioner to the hair ends and shafts without rubbing into the scalp or roots.
● Rinse hair thoroughly to remove excess product, which can cause dull hair.
● Wrap your head in a towel or turban and pat against your hair to absorb excess moisture. Don't rub vigorously, as this can ruffle or damage hair cuticles.
● Hold hairdryers at least six inches from your head. Dry the back and sides first, gradually reducing the speed and temperature settings as your hair dries. Stop while your hair is still damp and finish drying naturally.
● Choose heated rollers that are steam-producing and thermostatically controlled. Never sleep in rollers, pins or clips – this will damage your hair.
● Avoid uncovered elastic hairbands, which damage hair cuticles; use only thick, fabric-coated bands.
● Add a little argan, coconut, pumpkin seed or flaxseed oil to your hair (and to hairbands) to protect your hair and add shine.

★ *Top tip*

Choose a comb with widely spaced teeth and without mould lines down the centre of each tooth, which can damage hair shafts. If using a brush, select one with wide-spaced, plastic bristles that have smooth, blunt tips. Avoid combs and brushes with metal prongs.

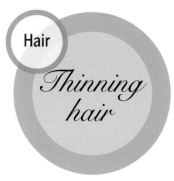

Thinning hair

What causes it? Thinning hair is linked with: age • menopause • post-pregnancy • physical or emotional trauma • lack of vitamin D, iron, zinc or other micronutrients • underactive thyroid gland

After the age of twenty-five the diameter of individual hairs naturally starts to decrease, and by the age of forty most people have finer hair with less body. At the same time, more follicles stay in their resting phase, resulting in progressive thinning.

➠ Falling oestrogen levels around the time of the menopause contribute to thinning hair, and a lack of vitamin D leads to disordered hair cycles and hair loss. Almost one in four women don't get enough iron to replace menstrual losses, and a further

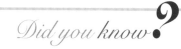

Did you know?

It's normal to lose a significant amount of hair after pregnancy, due to a fall in circulating growth factors and a synchronization of hair life cycles so they fall out at the same time. Within a year, hair has usually returned to normal.

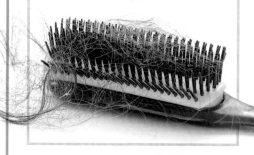

Lifestyle checklist

- Avoid excess stress.
- Stimulate the circulation to your scalp with a daily massage – simply take handfuls of hair and gently move the scalp to and fro, and side to side, to loosen tension and promote blood flow.
- Use a shampoo containing green tea caffeine, which blocks DHT production and stimulates hair growth. Caffeine also reduces smooth muscle constriction around hair follicles to improve blood flow and nutrient delivery. Just 2 minutes' contact with the scalp allows the caffeine to penetrate deeply, where it remains for up to 48 hours, even after hair-washing. Caffeine shampoos that also contain B vitamins can increase the cross-sectional area of scalp hair fibres by 10 per cent, to produce noticeable thickening.
- Ask your doctor to assess your thyroid function, and to measure your serum ferritin levels to look for iron deficiency.

one in ten don't get enough iodine; lack of either can lead to thinning hair.

Foods that can help

- **Eat more plant oestrogens.** Isoflavones are found in edamame beans and other soy products, sweet potato, lentils, nuts and seeds. Lignans have an additional beneficial action by inhibiting the enzyme 5-alpha reductase, which converts testosterone to the stronger dihydrotestosterone (DHT) in hair follicles. DHT increases male- and female-pattern hair loss.

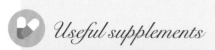

Useful supplements

Soy or **red clover isoflavones** provide phytoestrogens (probiotics increase conversion of soy isoflavones to a stronger version called equol)

Flaxseed oil is one of the richest dietary sources of lignans, which help with hair regeneration

Zinc helps to rebalance hair cycles; take within a multivitamin and mineral supplement to help to guard against deficiencies

L-lysine amino acid supplements are recommended by some nutritionists; l-lysine plays a part in the absorption of iron and zinc

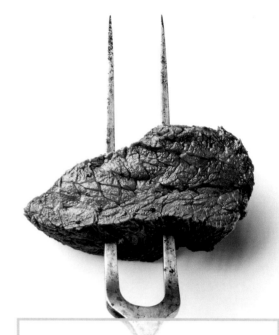

Researchers have found that high intakes of lignans (found in pumpkin seed oil, flaxseed oil, sweet potato) are associated with hair regeneration and a reduced rate of hair loss.

- **Grab some garlic** – it increases blood flow to hair follicles.
- **Increase intake of vitamin B$_{12}$,** which helps prevent loss of hair and is found in fish, eggs, chicken and milk.

NOTE: If you're a vegetarian, you need to ensure a good intake of the amino acid, lysine, vitamin B$_{12}$, iron and zinc.

Foods to avoid

- **Cut the salt!** Research shows that cutting salt intake can lessen hair loss by as much as 60 per cent.

SALON TECHNIQUES

- **Real hair** can be woven into your own hair to disguise patchy hair loss or thin panels; ask your hair salon for recommendations, or check online to find a specialist near you

Soy steak with pumpkin seed dressing

60 ml (2 fl oz) low-sodium soy sauce

1 tbsp Worcestershire sauce

zest and juice of 1 lemon

4 cloves garlic, crushed

freshly ground black pepper

4 lean steaks

TO GARNISH:
1 bag watercress (or other green leaves)

handful of pumpkin seeds

pumpkin seed or flaxseed oil (for drizzling)

Mix all the ingredients together and marinate the steaks for 30 minutes (or overnight in the fridge). Grill or pan fry the steaks to your liking and serve with watercress/green leaves, scattered with the pumpkin seeds and drizzled with pumpkin seed or flaxseed oil.

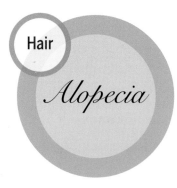

Alopecia

What causes it? **Alopecia is linked with:** abnormal white cell immune reactions within hair follicles • stress • lack of vitamin D • possibly iron deficiency • underactive thyroid

Alopecia is a common hair loss condition in which certain hair follicles stop growing. The exact cause is unknown, but it is thought to be due to an overactive immune system attacking the follicles. Vitamin D may be key in guarding against this distressing condition.

The most common form is alopecia areata, in which hair is lost in patches, usually on the scalp. Stress plays a major role, as it reduces blood supply to the scalp, and also seems to increase production of oily secretions by the sebaceous glands connected to each hair follicle. Vitamin D deficiency has recently been recognized as increasing the risk of alopecia.

Foods that can help

Because hair follicles are non-essential structures, if your body is deficient in nutrients they will be among the first to suffer – with nutrients diverted away from your hair. So try to adhere to the following guidelines:

- **Get a good intake of vitamin D** (found in oily fish, liver, eggs, butter, fortified milk and supplements) – this is essential.
- **Eat protein sources with every meal,** whether it's poultry, lean meat and fish or eggs, nuts and beans.
- **Eat plenty of wholegrains, fruit, vegetables and seeds:** these are a rich source of vitamins, minerals and essential fatty acids that hair roots need continuously.

Foods to avoid

- Avoid excess sugar, salted or processed foods.
- **Don't add salt to your food** during cooking or at the table.
- **Try cutting out certain foods:** some people have had success by cutting out animal foods and switching to a plant-based diet supplying protein from nuts, beans, wholegrains and seeds; others

Lifestyle checklist

- **Avoid excess stress,** which triggers abnormal immune reactions in the skin and causes blood vessels to constrict, reducing the flow of blood, oxygen and nutrients to your scalp.
- Obtain 15 minutes' sun exposure to your scalp two or three times a week.
- **Drink plenty of water** to improve the flow of nutrients.
- **Ask your doctor to assess your thyroid function,** and to measure your serum ferritin levels to look for iron deficiency.

Obtain 15 minutes' sun exposure to your scalp two or three times a week.

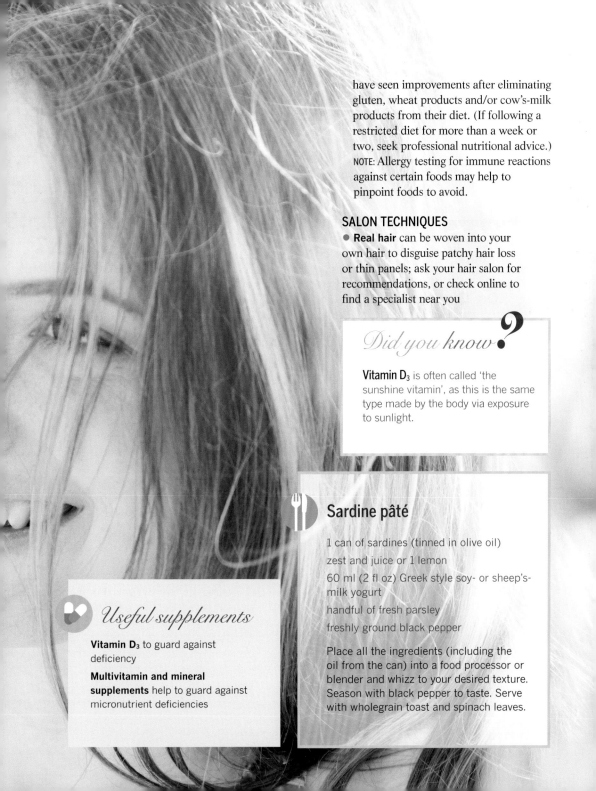

have seen improvements after eliminating gluten, wheat products and/or cow's-milk products from their diet. (If following a restricted diet for more than a week or two, seek professional nutritional advice.) NOTE: Allergy testing for immune reactions against certain foods may help to pinpoint foods to avoid.

SALON TECHNIQUES
● **Real hair** can be woven into your own hair to disguise patchy hair loss or thin panels; ask your hair salon for recommendations, or check online to find a specialist near you

Did you know?

Vitamin D₃ is often called 'the sunshine vitamin', as this is the same type made by the body via exposure to sunlight.

Sardine pâté

1 can of sardines (tinned in olive oil)

zest and juice or 1 lemon

60 ml (2 fl oz) Greek style soy- or sheep's-milk yogurt

handful of fresh parsley

freshly ground black pepper

Place all the ingredients (including the oil from the can) into a food processor or blender and whizz to your desired texture. Season with black pepper to taste. Serve with wholegrain toast and spinach leaves.

Useful supplements

Vitamin D₃ to guard against deficiency

Multivitamin and mineral supplements help to guard against micronutrient deficiencies

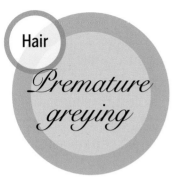

Hair

Premature greying

Hair colour – and the age at which your hair loses it – is genetically determined. If your hair is grey, some pigment is still present within the hair; if your hair is totally devoid of pigment, it becomes transparent and reflects light to appear snow white.

▶▶ Melanin-producing cells (melanocytes) at the base of each hair follicle feed pigments through to the hair root. If you produce red melanin you will have gold, auburn or red hair, while black melanin produces shades of brown or black, depending on its concentration. In blond hair, melanin pigment is pale and only found in the middle layer of the hair shaft (cortex). In dark hair, pigments are found in both the cortex and the inner core (medulla) to provide a greater depth of colour.

Hair turns grey due to an age-related decrease in the activity of tyrosinase, an enzyme that produces melanin from an amino acid called tyrosine. Some lucky people may

Useful supplements

Reishi extracts benefit circulation to improve hair health

Brewer's yeast is a good source of B vitamins and copper

retain their hair shade throughout life, but, for many women (an estimated one in three), colouring their hair is an essential part of their beauty routine. Chemicals found in hair dyes can irritate skin and cause allergic reactions, however, so it's a good idea to do a patch test first (the chemicals most commonly involved include PPD and other aniline dyes derived from coal tar, ammoniated mercury, lead and other toxic metals, as well as the bleaching agent peroxide).

Foods that can help

As premature greying of hair has been linked with a lack of certain vitamins and minerals, make sure you get plenty of the following, to give your hair colour a fighting chance:

- **Vitamin B₅** (also known as pantothenic acid or pantothenate) – found in wholegrains, beans such as edamame, lentils and beansprouts, vegetables such as broccoli, dark green leaves, avocado and tomatoes.

Lifestyle checklist

- Avoid excess stress, which can cause older, darker hair to fall out, so that younger grey hairs growing through seem more prominent. (This is the basis of the myth that hair can turn grey/white overnight!)
- Apply prune juice: this is traditionally used to cover a touch of grey, thanks to its rich, dark amber colour (see also page 53).
- See your doctor if also lacking in energy, to exclude an underactive thyroid gland.

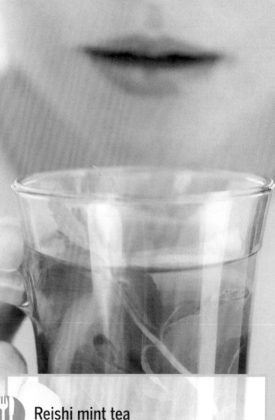

- **Vitamin B$_{12}$** – food sources include liver, kidney, oily fish (especially sardines), white fish, red meats, eggs and dairy products.
- **Folic acid** – found mainly in green leafy vegetables and wholegrains.
- **Copper** – obtained from seafood, nuts, beans, wholegrains, avocado, artichokes, radishes, garlic, mushrooms and green vegetables grown in copper-rich soil.
- **Reach for the reishi!** Dubbed the 'mushroom of immortality', this ancient Chinese remedy for premature hair-greying boosts blood flow to the peripheries and promotes the growth of healthy, glossy hair. It can be drunk as a tea.

Foods to avoid
- **Avoid processed convenience foods** and those with a lot of added salt – follow a wholefood, nutrient-rich diet instead.

SALON TECHNIQUES
- **Professional hair colouring** is offered by most hair salons. If possible:
- avoid man-made dyes and select the most gentle, natural products, such as herbal extracts (rosemary, cinchona, walnut husk)
- ensure dyes are kept away from direct contact with your scalp (using a skull cap or skilful application of colours)
- select paler shades (there are more chemicals in dark brown and black colours than in blond dyes)

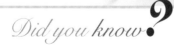

Did you know?

Blonds have more hairs than brunettes, but their hair is finer. Brunettes, in turn, have more follicles than redheads, and brown hairs tend to be thicker, giving a fuller look.

Reishi mint tea

3 g dried red reishi mushroom
1 handful fresh mint leaves
stevia or honey to taste

Infuse the reishi and fresh mint in hot water for 10 minutes. Sweeten with stevia or honey, as desired. (makes 1 cup)

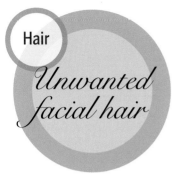

Unwanted facial hair

What causes it? Unwanted facial hair is linked with: genetics • age • menopause • hormone imbalances

The prevalence of unwanted facial hair increases with age as oestrogen levels decline, so give your levels a boost by increasing your intake of phytoestrogens – plant hormones found in beans, nuts, wholegrains and green leafy vegetables.

➤➤ Women usually start to notice a few stray, coarse hairs on the chin in their mid-forties, which slowly increase in number. By the age of sixty-five, 40 per cent of women also have noticeable hair above their upper lip. Some cases are linked with raised levels of circulating male hormones (such as testosterone, produced in excess in polycystic ovary syndrome), but up to a third of cases are simply age-related.

Lifestyle checklist

- **Pluck with good-quality tweezers,** if you only have a few coarse unwanted facial hairs (a magnifying mirror of x10 to x15 will make this easier).
- **Use a depilation cream** designed for use on the face, for dark hairs that are annoyingly visible rather than coarse; these can be dissolved every few weeks.
- **Avoid shaving hairs,** as this just cuts off the finer tips, so the thicker shaft grows back feeling 'stubbly'.
- **Seek medical advice** if hair growth seems profuse or is accompanied by acne, as you may need investigation and treatment for a hormonal imbalance.
- **Take regular exercise,** as this can improve hormone balance – but avoid over-exercising, which may make it worse.

As women approach the menopause, the amount of oestrogen released from the ovaries falls. Small amounts of a weaker oestrogen (oestrone) are still produced from the adrenal glands and body fat stores, however. Some testosterone is also produced from the adrenal glands, and the relative activity of testosterone compared with oestrogen increases. If your hair follicles are particularly sensitive to the effects of testosterone, facial hair growth may become troublesome.

The tendency towards facial hair is partially inherited, especially if you are of Mediterranean descent, or if you have dark hair, which makes it more noticeable.

Foods that can help

Increase your intake of isoflavones, flavonoids and lignans (oestrogen-like plant hormones) found in:
- **Beans** (especially lentils, alfalfa and mung beansprouts, chickpeas, edamame and other soy products)

Did you know?

In Japan, salons offer *kao sori* (shaved face), in which fine, downy cheek hair and dead skin cells are scraped from the face using a razor. This helps to promote a whiter, brighter, softer skin.

- **Vegetables** (especially dark green leafy vegetables such as broccoli, spinach, cabbage and kale, celery, fennel and exotic members of the cruciferous family like Chinese leaves and kohlrabi)
- **Nuts** (such as macadamias, almonds, cashews, hazelnuts, walnuts and nut oils)
- **Seeds** (especially flaxseed, pumpkin seed, sesame and sprouted seeds)
- **Wholegrains** (especially buckwheat, corn, millet, oats and rye)
- **Fruit** (especially apples, avocados, bananas, mangoes, papayas and rhubarb, plus dried fruits such as dates, figs, prunes and raisins)
- **Herbs** (especially angelica, chervil, chives, garlic, ginger, parsley, rosemary and sage)

Foods to avoid

- **Avoid excess sugar and saturated fat.**
- **Reduce salt intake** by avoiding obviously salty foods and not adding salt at the table or during cooking – use herbs for flavour instead.
- **Steer clear of alcohol and fizzy drinks.**

SALON TECHNIQUES

- **Laser therapy** can eliminate unwanted hair permanently, but between two and five treatment sessions, at four- to six-weekly intervals, are usually needed, as the laser energy only destroys hairs that are in their active growth phase. It works best on dark hair, as it is the dark pigment that absorbs laser energy and destroys the hair through a process known as photothermolysis. It does not work on blond or white hair.

Avocado, yogurt & beansprout salad

150 g (5 oz) plain Greek-style soy yogurt

handful of rocket leaves, chopped

handful of chives, chopped

250 g (9 oz) mixed beansprouts (such as mung, alfalfa, soy, radish, broccoli, lentil, red clover, quinoa, mustard, cress)

handful of nuts (such as macadamias, almonds, hazelnuts), chopped

large, ripe avocado, peeled, pitted and chopped

zest and juice of 1 lemon

good slug of pumpkin seed or flaxseed oil

freshly ground black pepper

TO SERVE:
dark green leaves of your choice

Gently toss all the salad ingredients together to combine. Season to taste, and serve piled on a bed of mixed, dark green leaves.

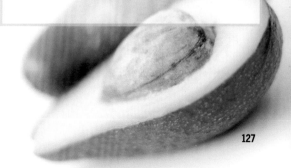

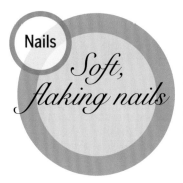

Nails

Soft, flaking nails

What causes it? Soft, flaking nails are linked with: genetic inheritance • lack of B vitamins, vitamins A and D, or silica • poor protein intake • lack of oestrogen at the menopause

Nails need a continuous flow of nutrients but, as non-essential structures, they often miss out when building blocks are diverted elsewhere during times of stress and poor diet. They are therefore one of the first parts of the body to show signs of nutritional deficiency.

▶▶ Nails are made of a tough, fibrous protein called keratin. Soft, thin, bendy nails that split and flake can result from an irregular supply of protein to your fingertips. One protein building block that is especially important is cystine, which helps to glue the keratin fibres together to increase nail hardness. Nails with poor water resistance soon soften when the hydration of the nail plate increases from the normal level of around 18 per cent to become greater than 25 per cent. Soft, flaking nails (hapalonychia) are also associated with low levels of magnesium and vitamins A and D.

Did you know?

Nails grow at a rate of around 5 mm (⅕ in) per month. Soft nails may grow more slowly.

Lifestyle checklist

- Apply wheatgerm, rosehip or macadamia nut oil to condition nails and improve water resistance.
- Avoid prolonged immersion of nails in water – use gloves when doing the dishes, and keep your hands out of the bath when enjoying a long soak.
- Exercise regularly to boost circulation to the nail beds.
- Avoid excess stress (and smoking), which constricts blood flow to nail beds.

Foods that can help

- **Include a protein source with every meal,** such as poultry, fish, lean meat and eggs – all of which are also good sources of vitamins A, B and D – or vegetarian sources, such as beans and nuts.
- **Munch macadamias:** these are especially good for your nails, as they provide a good amount of protein (10 per cent of their weight), including all the essential amino acids. Macadamia nut oil is rich in moisturizing monounsaturated fats and is included in many nail and cuticle oil formulas, as it rapidly sinks in.
- **Eat oily fish:** these are excellent sources of protein, vitamin D and omega-3 fatty acids which help to strengthen nails and add a glossy sheen.
- **Go for garlic** – it's a rich source of sulphurous amino acids, from which cystine is made.

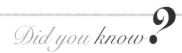

- **Seek out silica,** which increases cross-linking of proteins in the nail, improving their strength. It's found in nuts, seeds and a variety of vegetables, including beansprouts, which are also good sources of vitamins B_1, B_2, B_3 and folate, vital for rapidly dividing cells in the nail beds.

If thinning nails are associated with a lack of oestrogen after the menopause, eat more soy products such as edamame beans, tofu and miso soup. These provide a weak oestrogen boost that improves quality of skin structures, including the nails, as well as reducing hot flushes and night sweats.

Foods to avoid

- **Don't skip meals,** even when time is scarce, as a regular supply of protein and micronutrients is important for strong nail growth.

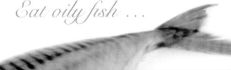

Eat oily fish ...

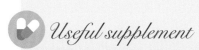

Useful supplement

Vitamin C is needed for production of collagen in the nail bed

B vitamins, including **biotin** (shown to increase nail thickness), are important for nail growth

Calcium may improve nail strength through effects on protein cross-linkage

Essential fatty acids (evening primrose oil, omega-3 fish oils) improve nail strength and water resistance

Soy isoflavones help to maintain oestrogen levels after the menopause

Soy lecithin is used to improve nail growth and strength

MSM (methylsulphonylmethane) supplies organic sulphur needed for keratin cross-linking

Reishi promotes growth of healthy, stronger nails

SALON TECHNIQUES

- **Seek advice from a nail technician** before taking action: although nails can be built up artificially with acrylics and gels, these can further damage soft, flaking nails

Fish salad with garlicky edamame & beansprouts

1 large carrot, peeled and grated

1 handful of shelled edamame beans

2 handfuls of beansprouts

200 g (7 oz) cold, cooked oily fish (eg mackerel, salmon, tuna, herring), flaked

FOR THE DRESSING:

2 tbsp rice wine vinegar

2 tbsp low-sodium Japanese soy sauce

2 tbsp apple juice

2 tbsp macadamia nut or olive oil

2 cloves garlic, crushed

Mix the carrot, edamame, beansprouts and fish together. Place the dressing ingredients in a screw-top jar and shake, then pour the dressing over the salad, toss well and serve. (If you like, add a chopped red chilli to spice things up!)

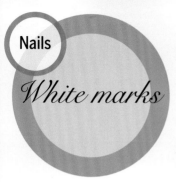

White marks

What causes it? White marks are linked with: trauma, especially if there is a protein deficiency, or lack of zinc or calcium in the diet

White spots frequently develop on nails. They may appear on just one or two, or all the nails may be affected. Occasionally, white bands may even form across the nail width. While not the sole cause, lack of zinc may be a contributing factor.

▶▶ There are numerous theories about the cause of white spots and streaks on the nails. Most popular is that they relate to minor unnoticed trauma (knocks and bangs) at the base of the nail, such as knocking a finger against a door frame. This was suggested because white spots are more frequent on the nails of the index and little finger of the dominant hand. However, similar spots also develop on the toenails, which are usually protected by footwear, so, although trauma is a factor, it is not the main or only cause.

In the 1950s, doctors noticed that low protein (albumen) blood levels could cause white banding by allowing fluid to leak

Drink plenty of water to improve the flow of nutrients to the nail beds.

Useful supplement

Zinc is important for growth and strength of nails

Vitamin C is needed for production of collagen in the nail bed

Biotin is important for nail growth and can thicken nails to improve their resistance to trauma

Calcium and **silica** improve nail strength through effects on protein cross-linkage.

Lifestyle checklist

- Avoid using your nails as tools!
- Remain alert for minor trauma to your nails, such as knocks and bangs.
- Drink plenty of water to improve the flow of nutrients to the nail beds.

from the circulation, compressing blood flow under the nails. In the 1970s, it was observed that zinc deficiency increased the chance of developing white spots by reducing the healing response to trauma. More recently, in 2004, it was reported that severely low calcium levels caused white banding on the nails due to arterial spasm, which responded to calcium treatment.

Severe protein or calcium deficiency is unlikely to be relevant for most people. Whether or not white marks on your nails are linked to low zinc levels remains controversial. If white spots are only present on a few nails, they are most likely to result from minor trauma to the nail bed; if they affect all nails, however, and cause a pattern of white bands across the width of the nails, you may well have a zinc deficiency.

Foods that can help

- **Bump up your zinc:** good dietary sources include red meat, seafood (especially oysters), liver, kidney, wholegrains, nuts, seeds (especially pumpkin seeds), pulses such as lentils and soy beans, eggs, sweet potatoes, beansprouts and yogurt.

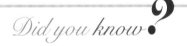

You can test for zinc deficiency by obtaining a solution of zinc sulphate (15 mg/5 ml) from a pharmacy. If the solution seems tasteless, zinc deficiency is likely; if it tastes furry, of minerals or slightly sweet, zinc levels are borderline; and if it tastes strongly unpleasant, zinc levels are normal.

Smoked oyster pâté

1 small can smoked oysters

1 small tub cream cheese

freshly ground black pepper

4 slices wholegrain toast

chives or parsley for garnish

Drain the oysters, then blend the oysters and cream cheese in a food processor. Season to taste. Serve spread on wholegrain toast, cut into wedges, garnished with the fresh herbs.

- **Eat a balanced diet** containing as many unrefined, wholefoods as possible: wholegrains, fruit, vegetables and seeds are a rich source of vitamins, minerals and essential fatty acids that provide nourishment for nail beds.
- **Eat a source of protein with every meal,** such as poultry, fish, eggs, nuts or beans.

Foods to avoid

- **Don't eat erratically or skip meals** (especially breakfast), or the supply of nutrients to non-essential tissues such as nail beds is reduced.

SALON TECHNIQUES

- **Professional manicures** will help to maintain nail condition; marks can be disguised with nail polish (bear in mind that excess pressure on the base of the nail may cause white spots to appear four to six weeks later as the new nail grows through)

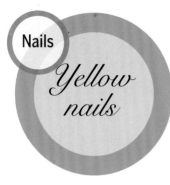

Nails

Yellow nails

What causes it? Yellow nails are linked with: using nail polish without a protective base coat • nicotine staining in smokers • fungal nail infections • poor lymph drainage and long-term lung disorders (rare)

The usual cause of yellow nails is applying nail polish without a base coat – and, in smokers, nicotine may be a factor, too. Increasing your intake of antioxidants affords your nails some extra protection.

▶▶ Nails are made of a tough protein called keratin, which is relatively transparent and colourless. The pinkness of healthy nails is due to blood flowing through tiny capillaries beneath. If nail polish is applied without a base coat, the pigments and chemicals within the polish quickly stain nails yellow, with darker shades having the most noticeable effect.

In smokers, nicotine can also stain the nails yellow, especially in those who do not use a filter. The best option, of course, is to quit smoking, although switching to electronic cigarettes and slowly cutting back will help.

If your nails are yellowed, roughened and thickened or crumbling, this suggests a fungal nail infection (see page 140).

Top tip

Lemon has a natural bleaching action that can clean some yellow stains from nails. Simply soak affected nails in a small bowl of fresh lemon juice for 15 minutes, then gently scrub with a soft nailbrush or old toothbrush. Apply macadamia, argan or wheatgerm oil afterwards to nourish the nails. Repeat daily. Another option is to scrub the affected area with a little whitening toothpaste.

Foods that can help

Foods that are rich in antioxidants may offer some protection to nails, especially fruits such as berries, mango, papaya, guava, cherries, prunes, pink grapefruit, pomegranate and red peppers. Antioxidants help to reduce the chemical reactions that can lead to discoloration within newly forming nail at the lunula – the crescent-shaped visible part of the nail root which produces new nail. The lunula is pronounced on the thumbnail but barely visible on that of the little finger. Nail growth starts from the root and grows upwards towards the tip of the finger, with additional nutrition supplied from the nail bed.

Foods to avoid

- **Tone down the turmeric:** it contains a powerful yellow pigment which may stain nails if handled frequently. Use ready-powdered root instead of grating your own.
- **Cut back on carrots:** though not harmful, eating excess amounts of carrot can stain skin and cuticles yellow-orange.

SALON TECHNIQUES

- **Professional manicures** will help to maintain nail health and appearance; ensure that a sufficient base coat is applied prior to polish, and remove polish regularly

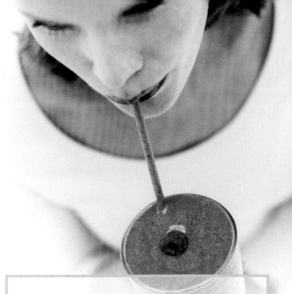

🍴 Berry smoothie

enough fresh or frozen berries (such as blackberries, raspberries, strawberries, blueberries) to half fill a 1 litre/4-cup blender jug

1 tbsp chia seeds

1 tbsp flaxseeds

2 tbsp honey

400 ml (14 fl oz) cranberry juice

Whizz all the ingredients together in a blender to obtain your desired consistency. Serve immediately. (You can add natural Greek yogurt if you prefer a milkier smoothie.)
(makes 4 small/2 large servings)

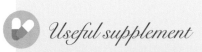

Useful supplement

Vitamin E (or applying a topical vitamin E oil) may help in some cases (vitamin E increases blood circulation and destroys free radicals that damage hair and nails)

Zinc is often recommended due to its role in maintaining nail health

Lifestyle checklist

- Always apply a base coat before painting your nails with a coloured nail polish; dark colours are the worst culprits.
- Try scrubbing the affected area with a little whitening toothpaste.

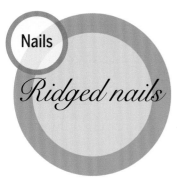

Nails

Ridged nails

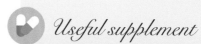

What causes it? Ridged nails are linked with: physical or emotional stress • exposure to excess cold or heat • irregular supply of protein or micronutrients, especially zinc

If nail growth is regular and continuous, the nail plate grows smoothly, but if growth is irregular or stops and starts, the nail plate becomes ridged. This is generally a result of stress or trauma affecting the supply of nutrients to your nails.

▶▶ Fingernails grow from base to tip, from the crescent-shaped lunula, over a six-month period, on average. Each month, you achieve a nail growth of around 5 mm (⅕ in) in length. Horizontal ridges that form bumpy waves across your nails are known as Beau's lines, and are due to a temporary stoppage of nail growth. These are a sign that you have experienced excessive stress – physical or emotional – over the previous few months. When you are stressed, the tiny blood vessels that supply nutrients to your nail beds constrict in response to stress hormones involved in the 'fight or flight' response. This is nature's way of diverting protein, vitamins, minerals and energy away from non-essential structures – your nails – and conserving them for use by your muscles and brain.

Useful supplement

Vitamin C is needed for production of collagen in the nail bed and is used up during times of stress

B vitamins, including **biotin** and **folic acid**, are important for nail growth

Zinc is important for growth and strength of nails

Co-enzyme Q10 improves oxygen uptake and energy production in cells

Garlic, **ginger** and/or **Ginkgo biloba** extracts help boost circulation to your nails if you have a tendency towards cold fingers

Lifestyle checklist

- Avoid excess stress and take time out for rest and relaxation.
- Get regular brisk exercise: this helps to burn off the adverse effects of stress hormones and boosts blood flow to your fingertips.
- Drink plenty of water to improve the flow of nutrients to the nail beds.

Did you know?

Ridged nails can result from anorexia (profound loss of appetite), due to low intakes of protein, vitamins and minerals.

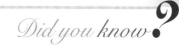

Vegetable spaghetti with tomato & pumpkin seed pesto

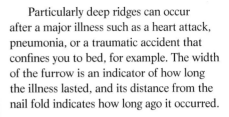

FOR THE SPAGHETTI:
1 large courgette
2 large carrots, peeled

FOR THE SAUCE:
12 semi-dried tomatoes
2 plum tomatoes, roughly chopped
handful of shelled pumpkin seeds
1 small bunch basil leaves
handful of rocket leaves
handful of baby spinach leaves
4 cloves garlic
4 tbsp freshly grated Parmesan
200 ml (7 fl oz) extra virgin olive oil
juice of 1 lemon

Using a spiralizer, make thin spaghetti-like noodles from the courgette and carrot. Add all the sauce ingredients to a food processor and pulse to make a paste. Place the vegetable spaghetti in a large serving bowl, drizzle with the pesto and gently toss to coat the spaghetti.

Particularly deep ridges can occur after a major illness such as a heart attack, pneumonia, or a traumatic accident that confines you to bed, for example. The width of the furrow is an indicator of how long the illness lasted, and its distance from the nail fold indicates how long ago it occurred.

Foods that can help

- **Eat a balanced diet** containing as many unrefined wholefoods as possible. Wholegrains, fruit, vegetables and seeds are a rich source of vitamins, minerals and essential fatty acids that provide nourishment for nail beds.
- **Go green:** green tea antioxidants have a general anti-ageing effect on the circulation, while the caffeine found in green tea dilates blood vessels to improve blood flow to the nails.
- **Top up on tomatoes:** these contain lycopene, which has a beneficial effect on the circulation.
- **Eat more garlic** – it dilates small blood vessels to improve blood flow to the nail folds by as much as 55 per cent.
- **Consume more zinc:** good sources include oily fish, beansprouts, lentils, sweet potato, edamame, green leaves, nuts and pumpkin seeds.

Foods to avoid

- **Don't eat erratically or skip meals** (especially breakfast), or the supply of nutrients to non-essential tissues such as nail beds is reduced.

SALON TECHNIQUES

- **Professional manicures** will help to disguise ridges by light buffing and application of a clear coat of protective lacquer

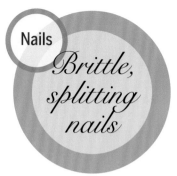

Brittle, splitting nails

What causes it? Brittle, splitting nails are linked with: heredity • menopause • underactive thyroid • low protein intake • lack of vitamin C, iron, zinc or silica • possibly gluten intolerance

Vertical splitting of the nails has been linked with lack of iron, zinc or silica, and is a sign of vitamin C deficiency. Poor hydration of the nail plate also leads to brittleness. So, if this problem affects you, it's time to adjust your diet.

▶▶ Brittle nails may seem hard and strong, but they break off before growing very long and split easily. Splits are sometimes horizontal but more often vertical. If the nail splits into the underlying quick, this can be intensely painful.

Foods that can help

- **Seek out silica,** needed to cross-link proteins in the nail, increasing their strength and overcoming brittleness. As well as strengthening nails, silica also improves skin elasticity and bone mineralization. Dietary sources include unrefined wholegrains, oatmeal, rice bran, green leafy vegetables, carrots, alfalfa beansprouts, nuts, seeds and cucumber rind.
- **Increase calcium intake:** calcium only makes up 0.2 per cent of the nail plate by weight, but contributes to nail strength through an effect on protein cross-linkage, so include dairy products in your diet.
- **Bring on the berries:** berries are an excellent source of vitamin C and bioflavonoids that improve collagen formation and help prevent brittle nails.
- **Eat more watercress,** which provides vitamins B, C and E – needed to build keratin.
- **Make it macadamias:** almost 10 per cent of their weight consists of protein, which, combined with their healthy oil content, makes them especially beneficial for brittle nails.

Foods to avoid

- **Try eliminating foods containing gluten** (wheat, rye, barley) for a month, to see if your brittle nails are linked with gluten intolerance. If this does help, seek advice from your doctor, who can arrange blood tests to confirm the diagnosis.

SALON TECHNIQUES

- **Specialist nail lacquer formulas** impregnated with protein, calcium and other substances are available, designed to reduce nail brittleness and splitting; ask your nail technician for details

Lifestyle checklist

- Drink plenty of water to improve flow of nutrients to your nail beds.
- Apply rosehip, argan or macadamia nut oil to strengthen nail plates, soften cuticles and improve water retention.

Did you know?

Iron supplements appear to decrease nail brittleness even in people who are not obviously iron-deficient.

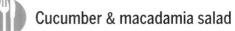

Cucumber & macadamia salad

1 cucumber, quartered lengthwise, then sliced (do not peel!)

200 ml (7 fl oz) natural Greek yogurt

handful of macadamia nuts, chopped

Mix all the ingredients together, and serve as an accompaniment to curries, cold meats and other salads.

Watercress provides vitamins B, C and E, needed to build keratin.

Useful supplement

Nail supplements containing silica from herbal sources, such as horsetail or bamboo, may be helpful

Biotin improves the strength of brittle nails by increasing nail thickness by at least a quarter (effects are usually seen within two to three months)

Essential fatty acids (evening primrose oil/omega-3 fish oils) improve nail quality, water retention, suppleness and sheen

Soy isoflavones help to maintain oestrogen levels after the menopause and can improve nail quality; these are best taken with a probiotic source (see also Edamame beans; pages 70–71)

MSM (methylsulphonylmethane) supplies organic sulphur needed for keratin cross-linking

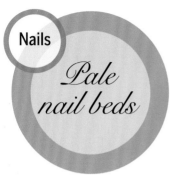

Nails

Pale nail beds

What causes it? Pale nail beds are linked with: anaemia (which can be nutritional, due to lack of iron, vitamin B_{12} or folic acid) • other causes include increased blood loss (heavy periods), reduced blood production (bone marrow suppression) or increased breakdown of blood (some autoimmune diseases)

Our nail beds should have a healthy pink tone, due to underlying blood vessels showing through the transparent nail plate. If pale, this could point to anaemia, which may have a nutritional cause.

➤➤ Our nails are made of a hard, fibrous protein called keratin. produced by active cells in the base and sides of each nail. These growing areas are protected by the cuticle skin folds. When red blood cells contain low levels of the red pigment haemoglobin, the resulting anaemia leads to pale nail beds and noticeable pallor inside the lower eyelids and lower lip.

If your nail beds look pale and you also feel tired and lacking in energy, it's important to tell your doctor. Anaemia always needs medical investigation to find out the cause. Nutritional causes include lack of dietary iron or folic acid, as well as poor absorption of vitamin B_{12}. Marked selenium deficiency, although rare, has been associated with a whitening of the nail plates, which quickly improves after taking selenium supplements. Severe lack of iron can also lead to brittle nails, and to thin, spoon-shaped nails (koilonychia).

Lifestyle checklist

• Avoid too much tea or coffee around mealtimes (coffee, for example, can reduce iron absorption by up to 39 per cent, if drunk within an hour of eating).

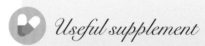

Useful supplement

Ferrous iron supplements (not ferric) are the recommended form: ferrous fumarate and ferrous gluconate are usually better tolerated than ferrous sulphate (wash down with freshly squeezed orange or berry juice)

Folic acid is essential for production of rapidly dividing cells in the nail bed

Co-enzyme Q10 improves oxygen uptake and energy production in cells

Foods that can help

• **Increase intake of iron-rich foods** if you're diagnosed with iron deficiency. Iron is most readily absorbed from the haem form found in red meats, but mineral iron is also available in bread, cereals such as oatmeal, pulses such as lentils and soy beans, egg yolk, green leafy vegetables (also a good source of folate) and dried fruit, especially prunes, cranberries and acai berries.
• **Combine plant sources of iron with vitamin C:** this more than doubles the amount of iron you absorb, so have freshly squeezed orange juice, berries, capsicum peppers or kiwi fruit, for example.

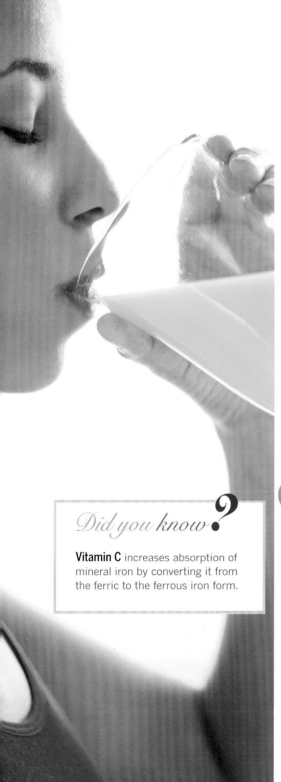

- **Bring on the Brazils!** Brazil nuts are the richest dietary source of antioxidant selenium, which is important for healthy nails.

Foods to avoid

- **Don't overcook veg:** over-boiling vegetables decreases their iron availability by up to 20 per cent, so eat them raw or only lightly steamed, where possible.
- **Avoid phytates** (found in most plant foods), fibre, calcium and tannin-containing drinks, as these decrease iron absorption.

SALON TECHNIQUES

- **Regular use of clear treatment lacquers is recommended;** if your nails are always painted with coloured varnish, paleness may not be detected

Did you know?

Vitamin C increases absorption of mineral iron by converting it from the ferric to the ferrous iron form.

Prune & Brazil nut compote

16 pitted prunes, halved

1 cinnamon stick

200 ml (7 fl oz) freshly squeezed orange juice

zest and juice of 1 lemon

2 tbsp honey

8 Brazil nuts, chopped

Soak the prunes and cinnamon stick in the orange juice overnight. Remove the cinnamon stick and discard, then add the remaining ingredients and stir well to combine. Serve cold or warm, as preferred (don't boil).

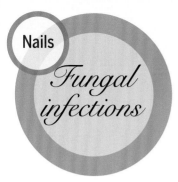

Fungal infections

What causes it? Fungal infections are linked with:

Trichophyton rubrum (the most common cause) – a fungus which also causes athlete's foot

Most fungal nail infections are preceded by a fungal skin infection such as athlete's foot. If left untreated, the fungus can spread into a nearby nail plate. While damaged nails cannot be repaired, you can take steps to ensure that new nail growth is healthy.

➡ When fungus spreads to a nail plate, it causes a localized patch of discoloured, roughened nail. If not addressed, this can progress to lift the nail from its underlying bed and can even lead to nail loss.

The aim of medical treatment is to protect new nail growing through. As your new nail plate develops it will look pink and healthy, compared to the scarred, discoloured end of the nail. Treatment must continue until the whole nail has grown through and been trimmed away, which can take three to twelve months. If treatment stops, the fungal infection usually takes hold again to invade any new, healthy nail growth you have achieved, so you have to start over again from the beginning.

Foods that can help

- **Increase intake of essential fatty acids** to help combat dry, damaged nails, as these are more easily infected.

Lifestyle checklist

- Sterilize nail clippers and scissors after each use to prevent spreading the infection to other nails.
- Always apply a base coat before nail polish.
- Don't bite or suck your nails.
- Avoid prolonged immersion of nails in water – always use gloves when washing the dishes.
- Have professional manicures to avoid damaging cuticles and nail folds.
- Massage coconut oil into hands and nails as a soothing, antifungal nail moisturizer.

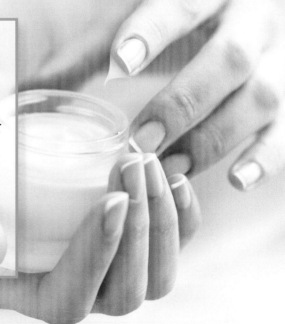

Massage coconut oil into hands and nails.

Did you know ?

Lemongrass, palmarosa, niaouli and red mandarin essential oils are more effective against *Trichophyton rubrum* than the traditionally used tea tree oil, according to research from the University of Derby, UK. Combining tea tree with lavender may increase its effectiveness.

Sources include oily fish (such as salmon, mackerel, sardines, herring and fresh tuna), as well as nuts and seeds.

- **Eat protein with every meal,** to boost keratin production – chicken, fish and eggs are good sources.
- **Grab some garlic:** it has a natural antifungal action, increases blood flow to the nail and contains sulphur, which promotes the formation of keratin to strengthen nails.
- **Go for ginger,** which stimulates circulation to boost blood flow to the nails.
- **Consume coconut oil:** it has a natural antifungal action and can be used in cooking – and is especially good for curries and stir-fries (see also page 24).

Foods to avoid

- **Cut back on sugary foods,** which are said to 'feed' fungal infections. (Although there's no conclusive evidence that this will help, it's good for your general health anyway.)

SALON TECHNIQUES

- **Laser treatment** can be effective for aggressive fungal nail infections – consult a qualified podiatrist

Coconut chicken stir-fry

a dollop of coconut oil

1 onion, sliced

4 chicken breasts, thinly sliced

a pack of tenderstem broccoli

2 tsp curry powder

1 x 400 ml (14 fl oz) can coconut milk

1 tbsp freshly grated ginger

1 pack fresh baby spinach leaves

coconut flakes for garnish

Stir-fry the onion and chicken in the coconut oil for 2 minutes. Add the broccoli and stir-fry for a further 3 minutes, then add the curry powder and stir-fry briefly before pouring in the coconut milk. Add the ginger and spinach, and cook until the spinach is just wilted. Garnish with coconut flakes.

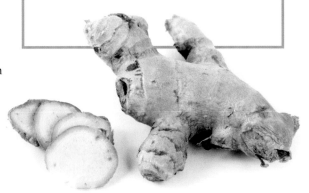

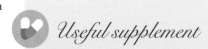 *Useful supplement*

Essential fatty acids (evening primrose oil/omega-3 fish oils) help to improve nail quality

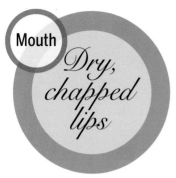

Dry, chapped lips

What causes it? Dry, chapped lips are linked with: exposure to harsh elements • licking lips • central heating • dehydration • lack of essential fatty acids • lack of iron, zinc or B group vitamins (especially B_2)

Repeated wetting and drying of the skin around the mouth is the main cause of dry, cracked or chapped lips, as this removes the natural, protective skin oils. Taking nutritional precautions can reduce your susceptibility.

Exposure to cold winds, a dry atmosphere in the home, licking your lips when stressed ... All of these contribute to chapped lips. Breathing through your mouth – especially at night – if you have nasal congestion is another common factor.

Nutritional deficiencies that increase the risk of developing chapped lips include lack of essential fatty acids, vitamin A and, if cracking affects the corners of the mouth, low iron or B vitamin levels.

Foods that can help

- **Drink sufficient water** to ensure you are not dehydrated. Sip water regularly – coconut water supplies useful additional nutrients.

- **Select orange-yellow fruit and veg** (such as mango, papaya, guava, carrots, sweet potato and pumpkin) for carotenoid pigments, which can be converted into vitamin A for skin healing. Dark green leaves are also a good source.
- **Increase intake of vitamin B_2** (riboflavin), found in wholegrains, eggs, dairy products, dark green leafy vegetables and beans such as edamame.

Foods to avoid

- **Don't over-boil veg!** Vitamin B_2 is readily lost into cooking water, to colour it yellow.
- **Don't leave milk bottles on the doorstep:** the riboflavin content of milk

Lifestyle checklist

- Use a humidifier in your home to help reduce dry skin, chapped lips and dry eyes.
- Use a protective lip salve, marigold ointment or calendula ointment on the lips regularly.
- Cover your lower face with a scarf when going out in cold windy weather.
- Apply slices of cucumber, or smear on a little honey, to help soothe dry lips.
- Avoid lip plumpers containing chilli if lips are cracked, chapped or sore.

Top tip

Coconut oil is a great balm for dry, chapped lips. Some lip salves now contain pomegranate, guava or mango for additional benefits (but avoid licking the delicious flavours!).

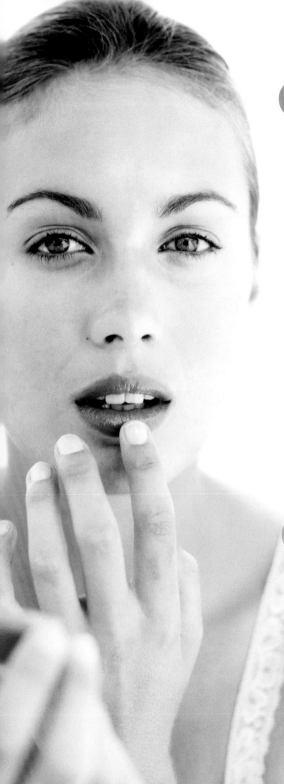

Coconut & watermelon smoothie

flesh of half a watermelon (deseeded)
500 ml (17 fl oz) coconut water
juice of 1 lime

Place all the ingredients in a blender and
whizz until smooth. Serve chilled.
(makes 4 small/2 large servings)

stored in clear bottles is reduced by
90 per cent after 2 hours' sun exposure,
so buy your milk in cartons, just to be
on the safe side.

- **Avoid freezing meat,** as this reduces its
vitamin B_2 content by up to 50 per cent.
Instead, try to eat fresh, organic meats
(also an excellent course of vitamin A,
iron and zinc).

SALON TECHNIQUES

- **Intensive lip moisturizers** can be applied
during a professional facial treatment

Useful supplement

Omega-3 fish oils, flaxseed oil or
evening primrose oil capsules supply
essential fatty acids (you can also
pierce a capsule containing evening
primrose oil and gently rub the oil
into your lips and surrounding skin
to soothe and protect)

Yeast extract is a good source of
B vitamins

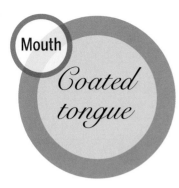

Coated tongue

What causes it? Coated tongue is linked with: dehydration • lack of dietary fibre • imbalance in mouth bacteria • poor digestive function

Does your tongue have an unsightly discoloured coating? This build-up of bacteria can be a sign of dehydration, or of a sluggish digestion with a tendency towards constipation and bad breath.

Foods that can help

- **Cram in the cranberries!** They contain unique substances known as A-type proanthocyanidins, which bind to certain bacteria and prevent them from sticking to the lining of the mouth and tongue. Drinking cranberry juice also helps to dislodge mouth bacteria from the tongue.
- **Drink sufficient fluids** (water, herbal teas, green tea) to prevent dehydration; green tea contains polyphenols with a natural deodorizing effect to suppress unpleasant odours created by mouth bacteria.
- **Follow a healthy, detox-style diet** with plenty of fresh fruit, vegetables, salads, soups and bio yogurt, plus beans and fish for protein.
- **Increase intake of fibre-rich foods** – most fruit and vegetables are good sources. Prunes are an especially rich fibre source, and can be soaked in green tea or light (reduced sugar) cranberry juice overnight, ready for breakfast. Bircher muesli, made by soaking oats, dried fruit, nuts (almonds or macadamias) and grated apple in apple juice overnight is another excellent fibre-packed start to the day.

Prune & cranberry smoothie

300 ml (½ pt) prune juice

300 ml (½ pt) light cranberry juice

handful of berries (cranberries, blueberries, blackberries) or pitted prunes

120 ml (4 fl oz) natural, unsweetened Greek bio yogurt

Place all the ingredients in a blender and whizz until smooth. Add additional cranberry juice or yogurt to obtain your preferred smoothie thickness. (If you prefer a juice drink rather than a smoothie, just leave out the fruit and yogurt.)

(makes 4 small/2 large servings)

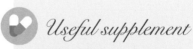

Useful supplement

Probiotic supplements provide 'friendly' digestive bacteria to help correct any intestinal imbalances

Milk thistle and **globe artichoke** supplements help to support liver function

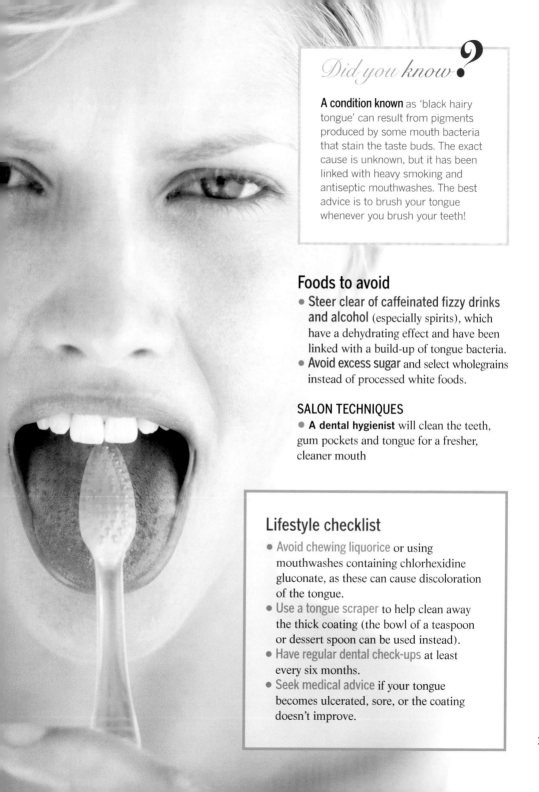

Foods to avoid

- **Steer clear of caffeinated fizzy drinks and alcohol** (especially spirits), which have a dehydrating effect and have been linked with a build-up of tongue bacteria.
- **Avoid excess sugar** and select wholegrains instead of processed white foods.

SALON TECHNIQUES

- **A dental hygienist** will clean the teeth, gum pockets and tongue for a fresher, cleaner mouth

Lifestyle checklist

- Avoid chewing liquorice or using mouthwashes containing chlorhexidine gluconate, as these can cause discoloration of the tongue.
- Use a tongue scraper to help clean away the thick coating (the bowl of a teaspoon or dessert spoon can be used instead).
- Have regular dental check-ups at least every six months.
- Seek medical advice if your tongue becomes ulcerated, sore, or the coating doesn't improve.

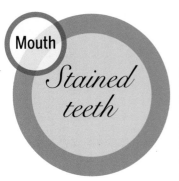

Stained teeth

What causes it? Stained teeth are linked with: staining with plant-derived pigments • smoking or chewing tobacco • side effects of some medications (such as fluorosis from excess fluoride during tooth development, or tetracycline antibiotics in early life) • age

Are you self-conscious about smiling for fear of displaying teeth that are less than pearly white? Teeth naturally become more yellow with age, and maintaining whiter, brighter teeth can have a dramatic anti-ageing effect.

Ironically, many of the antioxidants that give fruit and vegetables their beauty benefits and anti-ageing potential are intensely coloured pigments that can temporarily stain teeth. Rinse your mouth with water, green or white tea after eating intensely coloured berries.

Foods that can help

- **Choose cheese:** holding a piece of cheese in your mouth for a few minutes after eating fruit salad helps to neutralize the acid and supply a calcium boost.
- **Select fortified fruit juices** containing added calcium, as this decreases their erosive potential.
- **Boost calcium intake** with spinach and curly kale – both excellent sources.
- **Make a strawberry scrub:** strawberry can be used to remove stains from teeth – rub crushed fresh strawberry pulp directly onto your teeth, then rinse with plenty of water.

Foods to avoid

- **Watch your wine intake:** red wine is one of the worst culprits for staining teeth, as it contains high concentrations of chromogens and tannins, but white wine can also promote staining, due to its acidity.

Lifestyle checklist

- Practise good dental hygiene: brush twice a day, floss and/or use interdental brushes, as well as having regular six-monthly dental check-ups.
- Try white tooth 'paints', available from pharmacies.
- Rinse your mouth with a spoonful of coconut oil, swilling it around your teeth to help loosen stains.
- Use a straw to drink juices, unsweetened colas and iced teas (position the straw towards the back of your mouth and drink quickly, to lessen contact time with your teeth).
- Avoid brushing teeth for at least 30 minutes after consuming acidic food or drink – rinse with water instead.

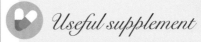

Useful supplement

Vitamin D is important for absorption of calcium from the gut

Co-enzyme Q10 helps to maintain healthy gums and, when combined with dental hygiene treatments, helps even receding gums to regenerate (recommended dose: 100 mg ubiquinol form daily)

Kale, Parmesan & macadamia salad with yogurt dressing

1 bag kale leaves, washed

handful of macadamia nuts, chopped

60 g (2 oz) Parmesan cheese, shaved

FOR THE DRESSING:
30 ml (1 fl oz) macadamia oil

zest of 1 lemon

1 tsp Dijon mustard

60 ml (2 fl oz) natural Greek-style yogurt

freshly ground black pepper

Trim the stalks from the kale and tear the leaves into bite-sized pieces. Plunge into boiling water for 30 seconds to soften, then plunge into cold water. Drain and place in a bowl. Top with the macadamia nuts and Parmesan cheese. Place the dressing ingredients in a screw-top jar, shake to mix, then drizzle over the salad. Season to taste.

Red wine is one of the worst culprits for staining teeth.

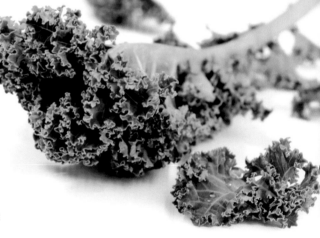

- **Steer clear of cola:** the acidity of fizzy colas damages teeth, and the brown pigments can become embedded in tooth enamel.
- **Avoid black tea** – the brown staining that builds up inside teapots and mugs can affect your tooth enamel, too. Drink green or white tea instead, as these contain fewer coloured compounds and tannins that can mark enamel.

SALON TECHNIQUES

- **Tooth-whitening treatments** are available, including bleaching procedures, bonding or the fitting of veneers; ask your dentist for advice

Did you know?

Mouthwashes can themselves cause discoloration of the mouth, especially those containing chlorhexidine, so try using warm green tea instead.

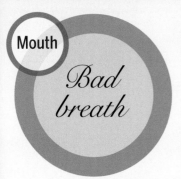

Mouth

Bad breath

What causes it? Bad breath is linked with: bacterial plaque • lack of saliva (dry mouth) • infection of the gums, sinuses, nose or lower respiratory system

Bad breath (halitosis) affects as many as eight in ten people at some time in their life and, while not a visible beauty issue, can destroy your self-confidence. Don't suffer in silence – there are steps you can take to help.

➡ Although popularly believed to result from a stomach or bowel problem, this actually accounts for fewer than 1 per cent of cases. The usual cause is a build-up of bacterial plaque in the mouth; these bacteria produce around 300 different gases and volatile chemicals, of which over 100 smell unpleasant.

Unfortunately, twice-daily cleaning of teeth is not usually enough to solve bad breath and gum disease, and mouthwashes are only a temporary solution.

Did you know?

People with gum disease are four times more likely to have bad breath. If your gums bleed when brushing, you may well have gingivitis (infected gums), which, if not treated, can lead to loss of teeth. Seek dental advice.

Lifestyle checklist

- Clean teeth twice a day, after eating.
- Use interdental brushes, dental tape or floss daily to clean awkward spaces between your teeth where rotting food and bacterial plaque lurk.
- Invest in an electric toothbrush designed to remove plaque efficiently; sonic versions that vibrate help to break up bacterial plaque.
- Chew gum containing xylitol, a natural sugar substitute that protects against tooth decay.
- Select a mouthwash that binds bacteria to remove them in visible clumps, or which oxidizes sulphur molecules to eliminate bad breath.

Foods that can help

- **Drink sufficient water** to maintain good hydration – usually around 2 litres (4 pints) per day in addition to the fluid naturally present in foods.
- **Stimulate saliva flow** first thing each morning by drinking a glass of citrus juice and eating two pieces of fruit, followed by thick, unsweetened, natural yogurt – Greek yogurt is ideal.
- **Drink green tea** – it contains polyphenols with a natural deodorizing effect to suppress unpleasant odours produced by mouth bacteria.
- **Eat calcium-rich foods,** such as yogurt and cheese, to help neutralize the acids found in fruit, juices and wine.
- **Chew peppermint or parsley leaves** to help mask mouth odours.

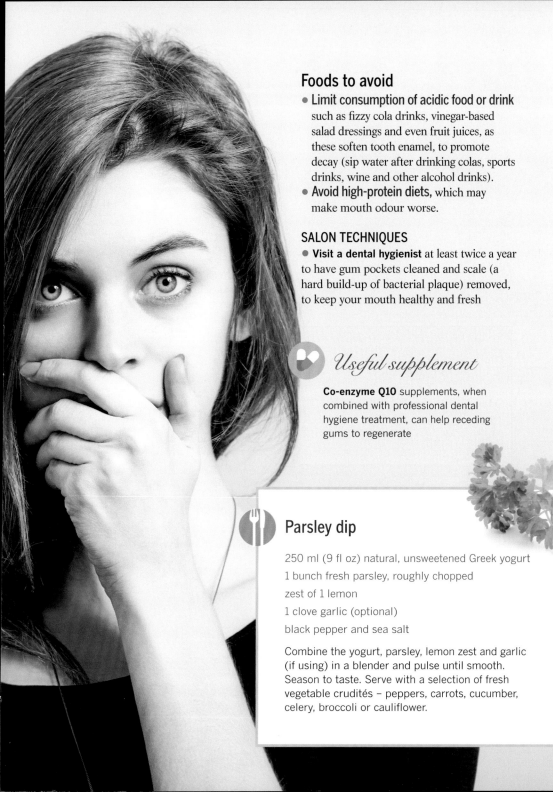

Foods to avoid

- **Limit consumption of acidic food or drink** such as fizzy cola drinks, vinegar-based salad dressings and even fruit juices, as these soften tooth enamel, to promote decay (sip water after drinking colas, sports drinks, wine and other alcohol drinks).
- **Avoid high-protein diets,** which may make mouth odour worse.

SALON TECHNIQUES

- **Visit a dental hygienist** at least twice a year to have gum pockets cleaned and scale (a hard build-up of bacterial plaque) removed, to keep your mouth healthy and fresh

Useful supplement

Co-enzyme Q10 supplements, when combined with professional dental hygiene treatment, can help receding gums to regenerate

Parsley dip

250 ml (9 fl oz) natural, unsweetened Greek yogurt

1 bunch fresh parsley, roughly chopped

zest of 1 lemon

1 clove garlic (optional)

black pepper and sea salt

Combine the yogurt, parsley, lemon zest and garlic (if using) in a blender and pulse until smooth. Season to taste. Serve with a selection of fresh vegetable crudités – peppers, carrots, cucumber, celery, broccoli or cauliflower.

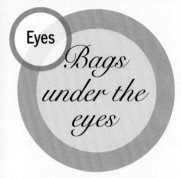

Bags under the eyes

What causes it? Bags under the eyes are linked with:
age • heavy sleep • fluid retention • wrong eye products

The delicate skin under the eyes is one of the first areas to lose its elasticity with age. As the density of collagen and elastin declines, there is an accompanying loss of moisture, suppleness and elasticity. Eating potassium-rich foods, and those that help reduce puffiness, can help.

➠ As the skin loses its ability to retain its shape and conform closely to the contours of the face, it starts to sag and accumulate fat cells to form a pouchy bag. When using skincare products under the eye, only use those designed for this texture of skin; creams that are too rich can lead to puffiness.

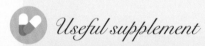

Useful supplement

Herbal remedies such as **dandelion** and **astragalus** have a mild diuretic action to reduce fluid retention

Acai & bilberry smoothie

ruby arils (seed pods) from 1 fresh pomegranate

100 g (3½ oz) frozen acai berry fruit puree (readily available online and in health stores)

small punnet of bilberries

1 banana, peeled

150 ml (¼ pt) unsweetened natural yogurt

500 ml (17 fl oz) coconut water

Put all the ingredients in a blender and whizz to obtain your desired texture.
(makes 4 small/2 large servings)

Puffiness also results from tiredness. During heavy sleep you produce more of an antidiuretic hormone designed to retain fluid (so you don't wake to visit the bathroom). This, together with the fact that you are lying flat (meaning any accumulated fluid does not readily drain away), also promotes puffiness beneath the eyes.

Foods that can help

- **Increase your potassium intake** by eating a wholefood diet with plenty of fresh fruit, vegetables, salads and wholegrains.

Get plenty of sleep!

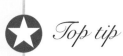
Potassium helps to flush excess sodium through the kidneys; sodium pulls water with it, to reduce fluid retention. Foods especially rich in potassium include seafood, tomatoes, bananas, pomegranate, pink grapefruit, prunes, sweet potatoes, pumpkin, carrots (raw), dark green leafy vegetables, edamame beans, yogurt, fresh juices and coconut water.

- **Drink acai juice** – traditionally used to reduce puffiness around the eyes (acai berry is commonly used in eye-skincare products, too).
- **Enjoy bilberries** – popular for promoting bright, healthy eyes and reducing puffiness.
- **Drink plenty of water** or herbal teas.

Foods to avoid

- **Cut back on carbohydrates** and follow a low-GI diet to reduce fluid retention.
- **Reduce salt intake,** as salt encourages fluid retention. Don't add salt during cooking or at the table – use herbs and black pepper for flavour instead – and avoid obviously salty foods. When salt is necessary, use potassium-enriched salts or sea salt sparingly.

Lifestyle checklist

- **Use an under-eye cream** designed to hydrate and tone the area, and apply sparingly.
- **Get plenty of sleep,** and ensure fresh air circulates at night by opening a window slightly (fit security locks if necessary).
- **Reduce puffiness** by sitting back, with your eyes closed, and holding a chilled spoon, chilled tea bags or thin slices of cucumber, sweet potato or strawberry over the eye area.
- **Use a small amount of macadamia nut oil** as a make-up remover, to cleanse the skin and gently melt away even the most stubborn mascara. As an additional benefit, it acts like a serum to sink in and nourish delicate skin around the eyes.
- **See your doctor** to have your blood pressure and, if necessary, kidney function checked, if puffiness lasts throughout the day.

SALON TECHNIQUES

- **Gentle, under-eye massage** can help drain fluid from the area through lymph channels; ask your beauty therapist for advice
- **Various surgical and non-surgical techniques** can reduce eye bags, including botulinum toxin injections, mesotherapy and blepharoplasty, to eliminate excess tissue under the eyes

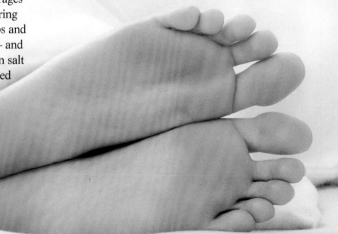

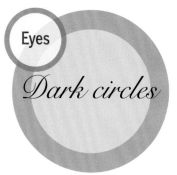

Eyes

Dark circles

What causes it? Dark circles under the eyes are linked with: heredity, tiredness and fatigue • hormonal imbalances • shadows due to ageing • dry skin, allergies/dermatitis • dehydration • nutritional deficiencies (especially of vitamins A, C, K, E and iron-deficiency anaemia)

Dark circles may appear for a number of reasons, but getting regular, refreshing sleep and taking steps to guard against nutritional deficiencies can help to resolve them.

▶▶ Dark rings under the eyes can be due to blood cells leaking from fine capillaries into the surrounding thin tissues, to cause bruising. This can occur due to fatigue and lack of sleep, especially if you keep rubbing your eyes to help stay awake. Allergies such as hayfever and skin conditions that promote rubbing of the eyes can also cause bruising.

More permanent dark circles may be due to a hereditary increase in pigmentation, hormone imbalances linked with pregnancy or oral contraceptives, anaemia, or from shadows cast when tissues in the eye area become more hollow with age.

Foods that can help

- **Eat a wholefood diet** with plenty of fresh fruit, vegetables, salads and wholegrains to ensure a good all-round intake of vitamins and minerals.
- **Increase iron intake** (if you have a deficiency) by eating meat, seafood (especially sardines), green leafy vegetables and dried fruit such as prunes.
- **Boost vitamin K,** needed to manufacture blood-clotting products, found in cauliflower, broccoli and dark green leafy vegetables such as spinach, yogurt (produced by the bacteria present), beansprouts, tomatoes and pulses such as edamame beans.

Lifestyle checklist

- Avoid excess facial exposure to the sun – use an under-eye product with a sun protection factor of at least SPF15.
- Apply chilled tea bags to your eyes – the cold and caffeine will stimulate circulation.
- Place thin slices of chilled tomato on your eyes, sit back and relax for 10 minutes (tomatoes have a natural bleaching effect).
- Gently apply coconut oil and pat into the under-eye area; leave on for a few hours, then remove with a cold cleanser.
- Use a cosmetic highlighter to disguise dark shadows.
- Sleep with fresh air circulating in the bedroom.

Did you know?

Thinning of tissues with age makes underlying blood vessels more visible and, at the same time, provides less support, so that leaking of blood cells, and bruising, is more frequent.

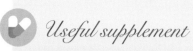

Useful supplement

A multivitamin and mineral will help to guard against micronutrient deficiencies

Pine bark extracts (Pycnogenol) help to strengthen tiny blood vessels and may reduce the tendency towards dark circles

- **Plump for pumpkin:** pumpkin seed extracts are rich in tryptophan – a building block for melatonin hormone, which helps to promote a good night's sleep.
- **Opt for argan oil** – also a useful natural source of melatonin, thereby helping to reduce dark circles.
- **Drink plenty of fluids** to avoid dehydration.

Foods to avoid

- **Cut out processed, convenience foods** and swap white bread, pasta and rice for brown versions to improve your intake of micronutrients.
- **Avoid excess alcohol and caffeinated products,** which will interfere with sleep.

SALON TECHNIQUES
- **Under-eye electrostimulant treatments** can boost circulation
- **Shallow laser therapy** or **microdermabrasion** can reduce pigmentation

Roast pumpkin puree with roasted seeds

1 small pumpkin
30 ml (1 fl oz) edible argan oil (or olive oil)
freshly ground black pepper

Preheat oven to 190°C/375°F/Gas 5. Slice off the stem end of the pumpkin and scrape out the seeds and membranes, reserving the seeds for toasting. Brush the argan oil inside the pumpkin, then bake in a shallow pan for 45 minutes to an hour, or until the pulp is tender. Meanwhile, wash the pumpkin seeds in a bowl of cold water and remove any remaining pulp. Pat seeds dry with kitchen paper and toss in a bowl with a little argan (or olive) oil to coat them well. Spread out on a baking sheet and roast in the oven for the final 30 minutes of the pumpkin cooking time. (You can flavour the seeds by adding black pepper, paprika, garlic or dried herbs with the oil, if preferred.)

Drain any accumulated liquid from the pumpkin, scoop out the pumpkin pulp and mash. Season to taste. Serve sprinkled with the roast pumpkin seeds.

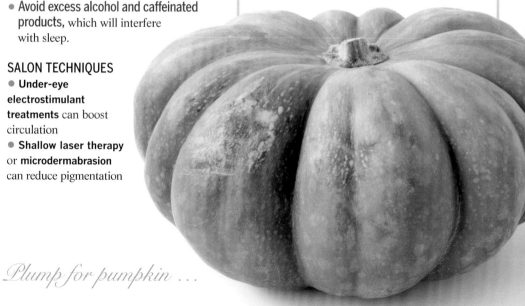

Plump for pumpkin …

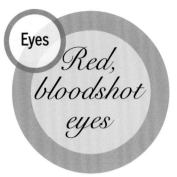

Red, bloodshot eyes

What causes it? Red, bloodshot eyes are linked with: dry eyes • allergies – especially to contact lens fluids • chemical irritation (such as chlorine in swimming pools) • eye fatigue • lack of sleep • conjunctivitis

Redness of the eye is due to dilation of blood vessels in the eye white; other causes include chemical irritation or allergic reactions and dryness due to reduced tear production. Boosting your intake of omega-3s can help to reduce inflammation.

▶▶ When concentrating on your work, you may not blink as frequently as normal, leading to dryness and feelings of grittiness and tired eyes, especially at the end of a long day in front of a computer screen. Redness in one eye, due to a bleed from a broken blood vessel (subconjunctival haemorrhage) can look dramatic but is usually harmless and disappears within a week or two. It's worth having your blood pressure checked, however, and try to avoid rubbing your eyes. (If redness is accompanied by soreness or pain, seek medical advice to rule out infection or an eye condition needing urgent treatment.)

Blepharitis, an inflammation of the eyelids, can be due to an allergic reaction to cosmetics, face creams, perfume, shampoo or even nail varnish. Stop using your usual products, then gradually reintroduce them, one at a time, to see if any retrigger the problem.

Foods that can help

- **Increase intake of omega-3s,** as the oils help to reduce inflammation. Good sources include oily fish such as sardines, seeds (especially pumpkin and flaxseed) and nuts (especially walnuts). Drizzle flaxseed or pumpkin seed oil over vegetables and salads.
- **Make it monounsaturated:** avocado

Lifestyle checklist

- Take regular screen breaks every 20 minutes, if you work with a computer.
- Remember to blink! – a common cause of dryness and grittiness when concentrating.
- Use lubricating eye drops (artificial tears) or a lubricating mist that you spray onto closed eyelids.
- Avoid rubbing eyes when preparing foods – especially chillies! Pungent onions can cause eye watering (put the chopped pieces in a bowl of water to help minimize this). You can also wear 'onion goggles' during preparation.
- Seek immediate medical advice if eyes are sore or vision is affected.

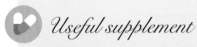

Useful supplement

Evening primrose oil and/or **omega-3 fish oil** supplements can help to reduce dry eyes, especially in contact lens wearers

Bilberry pigments help to stabilize tear production

Sea buckthorn oil is a traditional oral treatment for dry eyes

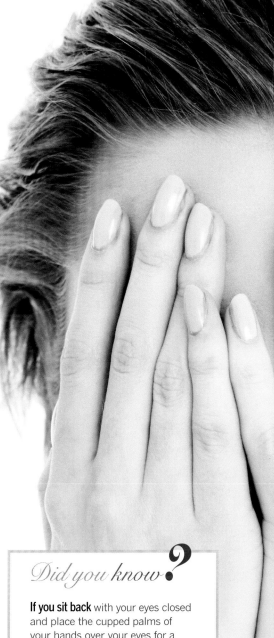

Sardine, avocado & flaxseed toasties

1 can of sardines in oil

1 avocado, peeled and pitted

zest and juice of 1 lime

1 tsp chopped red chilli (optional)

freshly ground black pepper

4 slices wholegrain toast

handful of rocket leaves

flaxseed oil for drizzling

Mash together the sardines in oil, avocado, lime and chilli (if using), and season to taste. Pile the mixture onto slices of wholegrain toast, and serve with rocket leaves and a drizzle of flaxseed oil.

(makes 4 small or 2 large servings)

and macadamia nuts, plus their oils, supply monounsaturated fats that are beneficial for dry eyes.

● **Drink plenty of fluids** to reduce inflammation – water, juices and herbal teas are ideal.

SALON TECHNIQUES

● **See an optometrist** for an eye check-up, in case you need glasses or a different prescription

● **Beauty specialists** can offer tips on using cosmetics to minimize redness (such as using a flesh-coloured eyeliner on the lower inside lash line – as long as your eyes are not inflamed – or a neutral-coloured eyeshadow to brighten eyes)

Did you know?

If you sit back with your eyes closed and place the cupped palms of your hands over your eyes for a few minutes, your eyes will feel remarkably refreshed when you move your hands away.

FURTHER READING
Other recommended titles by Dr Sarah Brewer

Arthritis for Dummies, Wiley, 2006

Cut Your Cholesterol, Quercus, 2009

Cut Your Stress, Quercus, 2010

Death: A Survival Guide, Quercus, 2011

Essential Guide to Vitamins, Minerals and Herbal Supplements, Right Way, 2010

The Human Body, Quercus, 2009

Intimate Relations: Living and Loving in Later Life, Age Concern, 2004

Live Longer Look Younger, Connections Book Publishing, 2012

Low-Cholesterol Cookbook for Dummies, Wiley, 2009

Menopause for Dummies, Wiley, 2007

Natural Approaches to Diabetes, Piatkus, 2005

Natural Health Guru: Overcoming Arthritis, Duncan Baird, 2009

Natural Health Guru: Overcoming Asthma, Duncan Baird, 2009

Natural Health Guru: Overcoming Diabetes, Duncan Baird, 2008

Natural Health Guru: Overcoming High Blood Pressure, Duncan Baird, 2008

Thyroid for Dummies, Wiley, 2006

The Total Detox Plan, Carlton, 2000, 2011

INDEX

picture credits

Cover MariuszBlach/Thinkstock
Supplements logo (repeats throughout): Naatali/ShutterStockphoto,Inc
Apple logo (repeats throughout): Kanate/ShutterStockphoto,Inc

Thinkstock 2–3 MariuszBlach; 3 Yuri; 5 monkeybusinessimages; 6–7 Ingram
Publishing; 8–9 Stockbyte; 10–11 Brand X Pictures; 12–13 Izf; 14–15 Viktar;
16–17 Jupiterimages; 18–19 Stockbyte; 20 ariwasabi; 22–23 luisapuccini;
23 Purestock; 24–25 Digital Vision; 26 aodaodaodaod; 27 Stockbyte;
28–9 Ekkapon; 29 Ingram Publishing; 30 unalozmen; 31 ElrondPeredhil;
32 Tatiana Belova; 33 esp2k; 34 JOHANWILKE; 34–35 George Doyle; 37
Stockbyte; 38 Digital Vision; 39 Stockbyte; 40 AbbieImages; 41 Stockbyte;
43 Stolensun; 44 Franck-Boston; 44–45 Stockbyte; 46 Stockbyte; 47
icenando; 48 jlbuyz; 49 siwaporn999; 50 Mark_Hubskyi; 51 NatashaPhoto;
52 Tuned_In; 53 nata_vkusidey; 54 Martin Poole; 55 piotr_pabijan;
56t Will Heap; 56b AlekZotoff; 57 Will Heap; 59 Peter Zijlstra; 61 Digital
Vision.; 62 Stockbyte; 63 manyakotic; 65 Lecic; 67 gresei; 68 franny-
anne; 70 Torsakarin; 71 Jimejume; 72 nata_vkusidey; 73 George Doyle; 74
shawn_hempel; 75 George Doyle; 76 Stepan Popov; 77 VladimirFLoyd; 78
moodboard; 80 gibgalich; 81 YekoPhotoStudio; 82 Thomas Northcut; 83
MIMOHE; 84 robynleigh; 85 Jupiterimages; 86 Magone; 87 Goodshoot; 88
Jupiterimages; 90 Lisovskaya; 91 Pixland; 93 Jupiterimages; 95 Flamingo_
Photography; 97 Secha6271; 98 Valeriya; 99 LuminaStock; 100 Stockbyte;
101 Buriy; 104 chengyuzheng; 105 Goodshoot; 106 AndrisTkachenko; 107
supercat67; 109 Purestock; 111 Jupiterimages; 113 naponfxhimorning; 114
RoborDestrani; 115 robynmac; 116 SonerCdem; 117 Pixland; 119 Stockbyte;
120 pan38; 121 Lisovskaya; 122–123 lorenzoantonucci; 125 George Doyle;
126 EdnaM; 127 Stockbyte; 128–129 Azure-Dragon; 130 Stockbyte; 131
Arijuhani; 132 Laurent Hamels; 133 Stockbyte; 138-139 tetmc; 139 Riverlim;
140 Ridofranz; 141 Sensay; 142–143 Stockbyte; 144-145 George Doyle; 146
donfiore; 147 robynmac; 149 MayerKleinostheim; 150–1 AndreyPopov; 152
IgorDutina; 153 Will Heap; 154–5 sonatali; 155 macniak

ShutterStockphoto,Inc 60–61 Boris Franz; 60 mama_mia; 66 Pairoj
Sroyngern; 103 Daxiao Productions; 134–135 thefoodphotographer;
137 Quang Ho; 148-9 file404

iStockphoto 42 Brasil2; 58 NRedmond; 69 gerenme; 79 MarkGillow

acknowledgements

I would like to thank everyone who has been
so helpful in providing research papers and
information for the insights explored in this book.

eddison books limited

Publishing Consultant Nick Eddison
Managing Editor Tessa Monina
Proofreader Nikky Twyman
Indexer Marie Lorimer
Design Jane McKenna (www.fogdog.co.uk)
Production Sarah Rooney